Prescription for Health and Long Life:

A Dose of Common Sense

By Shawn Konecni, PhD

Printed in the United States of America

First Printing, 2015

ISBN-13: 978-0-9913191-1-4

Breakout Concepts LLC

Contact – bcinfo@breakoutconcepts.com

Disclaimer

The information presented in this book is intended for informational and educational purposes only. The author and publisher have made every effort to ensure that the information contained herein is as accurate as possible at the time of writing. It cannot contain all of the information available on any one subject and some of the information may not be up-to-date. As such, the information is provided on an as-is basis. Any errors or omissions, whether typographical or in content, are unintentional.

Furthermore, this book should not be used as a substitute for professional medical advice. You should not use this information to diagnose or treat any medical condition. Consult your healthcare provider before starting any diet or exercise program, before taking any medication, or if you suspect you have any health problem. Any use or misuse of the information contained in this book is solely the responsibility of the user.

To my dad,

Without his encouragement and support, I would not have been able to finish this book.

Table of Contents

Introduction...1

Information Overload..1

Leading Causes of Death and Disability................................2

The Vicious Circle of Chronic Disease...................................4

Risk Factors of Chronic Disease..6

A Common Sense Approach to Health and Longevity..........10

How This Book is organized..11

Chapter 1: Diet and Nutrition...15

The Importance of Diet and Nutrition....................................15

What Makes a Healthy Diet?...16

Diet Plans for Health 18

General Recommendations for Weight Loss.........................20

Alternative Sources of Nutrition..24

Dietary Sources of Nutrients 28

Herbal Supplements..33

Putting it All Together 35

Chapter 2: At the Grocery Store 37

Shopping for the Right Food...37

The Nutrition Facts Label 39

Functional Foods 42

Product Marketing Labels 44

Factors that Influence the Nutritional Quality of Food 49

Food Additives and Health 52

Chemical Contamination in Food 56

Putting it All Together 59

Chapter 3: Kitchen Basics **63**

Food Preparation and Health 63

Preventing Nutrient Loss during Processing....................65

Preventing Nutrient Loss during Storage 68

Chemical Contamination in Food 72

Biological Contamination in Food 78

Putting it All Together 80

Chapter 4: Exercise and Physical Activity.................**83**

The Importance of Exercise and Physical Activity 83

Aerobic Exercise 85

Strength Training...92

Other Physical Activities..93

Lifestyle-Related Physical Activities 96

Putting it all Together..97

Chapter 5: Sleep and Stress Management **99**

The Dangers of Lack of Sleep and Excessive Stress 99

How Much Sleep Do You Need?...................................101

Factors that Can Affect Quality of Sleep 102

Guidelines for Better Sleep 104

Recognizing the Signs of Stress 109

Remedies for Mitigating Stress 111

Putting it all Together..115

Chapter 6: Environmental Chemical Hazards **119**

Chemical Exposure and Health.....................................119

Household Chemicals 120

Building Materials and Furnishings 125

Indoor Air Pollution 126

Outdoor Air Pollution 129

Water Pollution 131

Chemicals in the Garden 132

Putting in All Together..133

Chapter 7: Biological Pollutants and Germs 135

Biological Contamination in the Environment 135

Common Biological Pollutants and Germs 137

Control Measures Inside and Outside the Home 139

When All Else Fails..152

Sexually Transmitted Infections and Long-Term Health 154

Putting it All Together 154

Chapter 8: Technology Related Health Hazards 157

The Potential Dangers of Modern Technology........................157

Effects of Radiation from Electromagnetic Fields 159

How to Reduce EMF Exposure 162

Preventing Neck and Back Problems......................................165

Putting it All Together 169

Chapter 9: Cosmetics and Skin Protection 171

Protecting Your Skin 171

Signs of Skin Irritation 173

Contamination of Cosmetics and Personal Care Products.....174

Reducing Chemical Exposure 177

Chemicals in Clothing 179

Reducing Ultraviolet Radiation Exposure 180

Tattoos and Long-Term Health...182

Hand Sanitizers and Antibacterial Soaps...............................183

Putting it All Together 185

Conclusion **187**

Bibliography **193**

Introduction

Information Overload

When it comes to health, most of us would probably like to live a long time. More importantly, most of us would like to enjoy a high quality of life for as long as possible. What stands in our way? Bad habits, poor nutrition, dirty air, diseases, and even bad luck threaten to cut us off early or make our lives miserable. Surely there has to be something we can do about it other than simply going to the emergency room when we are sick.

Luckily, there are a number of preventive actions we can take to improve our health and live longer, all on our own. So, it seems all we have to do is find the right authority on the matter and do what they suggest is effective for our own lives. Of course, this is easier said than done.

We live in a world where authoritative information is flying at us from every direction and from every corner of the earth. Yet, it seems like it is getting harder and harder to identify what works and what doesn't. Why all the confusion? It turns out that modern technology both helps and hinders our quest for the truth. We are treated every day to an endless buffet of websites, blogs, news articles, social media content, and scientific journals. The list goes on and on. And that is in addition to all the advice from a number of self-proclaimed experts we run into every day at home, school, and work. Our doctors tell us one thing, and then the celebrities on television, some of whom may also be doctors, tell us something different. The inevitable result of all this mayhem is that many of us shrug our shoulders and go on with our lives, convinced that there probably isn't a convenient answer to anything and that it is easier to just wait until our number comes up in life's lottery. From there, we may either be forced to take action when it is too late, or perhaps be forced to check into a hospital.

There has to be a better way.

Introduction

One of the goals of this book is to help sift through this deluge of information in order to discern what is most important to maintain health. We will identify common sense actions to improve our lives over the long-term and increase our lifespan. We will also ensure that what we do makes sense in the modern world with the greatest chance of actually working, as opposed to just being fashionable. We need to leave blind experimentation up to the laboratory mice.

There is no time to waste, so let's get started.

Leading Causes of Death and Disability

So, what are we actually dealing with here? When discussing health and longevity, we need to understand what conditions are most likely to undercut our efforts as we age. A good starting point is to look at recent data indicating the leading causes of death in the United States (figure 1) [1].

You'll notice that most of these causes are related to chronic diseases such as heart disease, cancer, respiratory disease, and diabetes. Chronic diseases are defined as diseases that persist for an extended period of time. By an extended period of time, we mean months to years. They are not short-term conditions, also known as acute conditions, that come and go like a common cold. As illustrated, chronic diseases are responsible for most of the deaths in the United States. Other causes of death, such as severe injuries from accidents, are often related to chronic disease conditions that weaken the body over time.

As we age, we can expect our chronic disease risk to increase. We can also expect a higher risk for certain debilitating conditions and disabilities. These conditions can make people even more susceptible to long-term health problems as a result of physical inactivity and other complications. Table 1 lists some of the most common causes of disability in the United States [2].

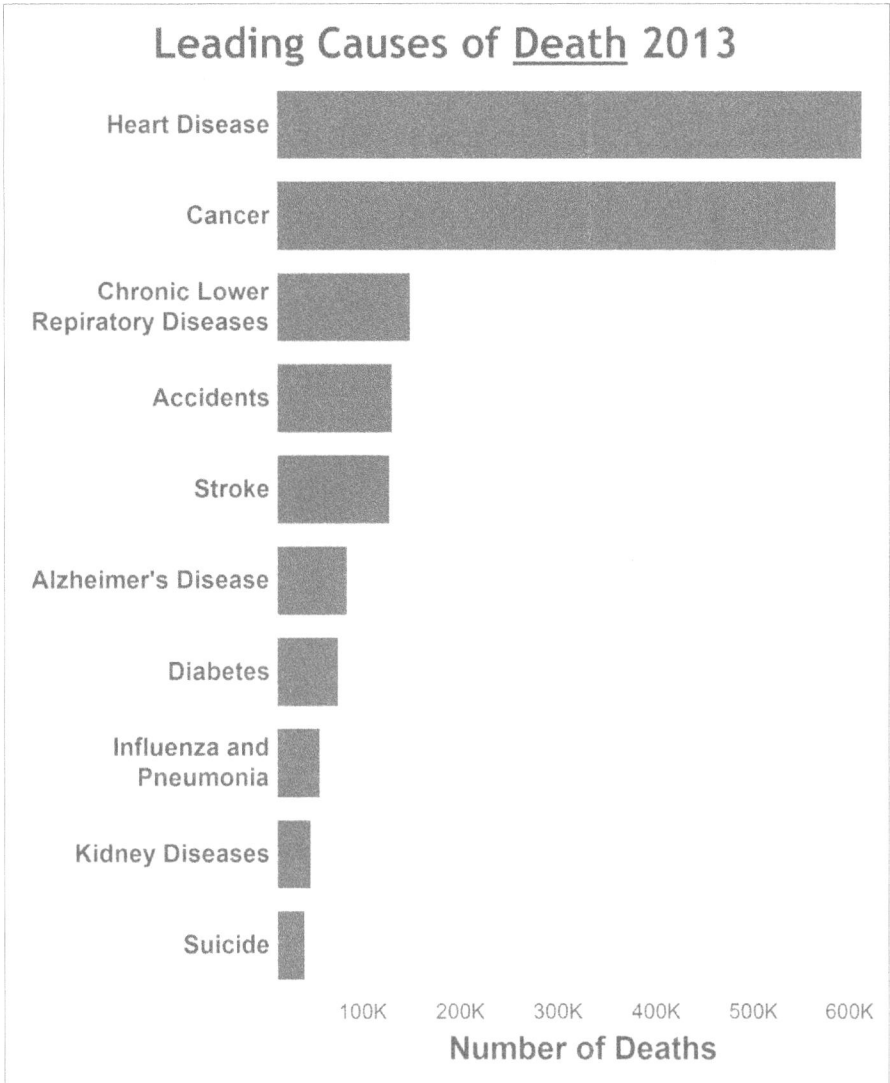

Figure 1 – Leading causes of __death__ in the United States. Chronic diseases are responsible for most of the deaths. Other causes of death are often related to chronic disease conditions that weaken the body over time.

Arthritis or rheumatism	Deafness or hearing problem	High blood pressure
Back or spine problem	Stiffness or deformity of limbs or extremities	Senility, Dementia, or Alzheimer's disease
Heart trouble	Blindness or vision problem	Head or spinal injury
Lung or respiratory problem	Stroke	Kidney problem
Mental or emotional problem	Cancer	Stomach or digestive problem
Diabetes	Broken bone or fracture	Paralysis

Table 1 – Common causes of <u>disability</u> in the United States. Disabilities are largely influenced by chronic diseases.

It is important to note that such disabilities are largely influenced by chronic diseases. Furthermore, as both mobility and functional capability decrease, we potentially trigger other chronic conditions in turn.

The Vicious Circle of Chronic Disease

One could look at the relationships between chronic diseases and disabilities as a vicious circle (figure 2) [3, 4]. In reference to overall health, once we enter this circle, it is difficult to get out of it, and it is easy to develop other associated conditions. As we accumulate more chronic conditions, we essentially accelerate our degenerative state.

Therefore, it is not enough to focus on any one chronic disease or disability when it comes to long-term health. The interrelated nature of chronic diseases and disabilities means that experiencing one problem could lead to a chain reaction.

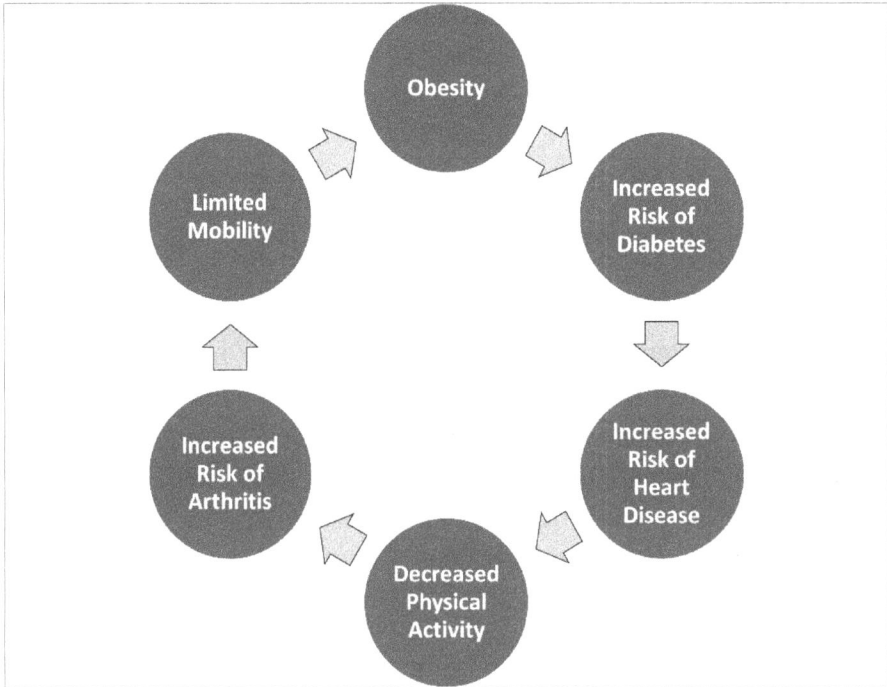

Figure 2 – An illustration of the vicious circle of chronic disease and disability. Chronic disease conditions often lead to other chronic diseases and disabilities. In reference to overall health, once we enter this circle, it is difficult to get out of it.

Of course, if you are already suffering from one of these conditions, you will still have recourse through the methods introduced in this book. It simply means you will have to redouble your efforts to stay healthy.

To deal with this multifaceted threat, we need a comprehensive preventive strategy that addresses all chronic diseases and conditions simultaneously. This goes for everyone, regardless of the fact that we are all different genetically. Naturally, a condition that causes a chronic disease in one person may not affect the next. Keep in mind, however, that chronic diseases tend to be interrelated. Even the symptoms themselves could trigger other chronic diseases in individuals who feel safe otherwise.

The bottom line is that it often takes only one medical or health problem to enter the vicious circle of chronic disease. But, there are things you can do to avoid this scenario.

Risk Factors of Chronic Disease

The association between chronic diseases and other conditions can be traced back to common risk factors in humans. A risk factor is essentially any condition that increases the likelihood of developing a disease or disability. Some of them are well-known, while others are largely ignored as problems that should only be addressed by the elderly population. Unfortunately, unresolved risk factors can make anyone, at any age, more susceptible to chronic disease over time. Therefore, it is a mistake to ignore them at any point in our lives.

Some of the risk factors can be mitigated by simply changing our behavior or manipulating our immediate environment. Others are the result of traits inherited when we are born.

The following risk factors **can be controlled or modified** through changes in behavior or manipulation of our local environment.

● **Poor diet and inadequate nutrition** – The foods we consume dramatically impact our overall health. Nutritional deficiencies caused by a poor diet can increase the risk of chronic disease across the board.

● **Physical inactivity** – An inactive lifestyle increases the risk of numerous chronic diseases and other debilitating conditions including heart disease, stroke, kidney disease, arthritis, and osteoporosis (bone disease) [5]. Additionally, weight gain from the same level of inactivity can lead to obesity.

● **Obesity** – Unhealthy weight gain is directly associated with a number of chronic diseases and conditions including heart disease, stroke, high blood pressure, type 2 diabetes, cancer, respiratory problems, sleep disorders, arthritis, and mental health problems [6]. This is one of the most important risk factors as it has an almost universal effect on mortality. An obese person is liable to experience a myriad of associated health complications at the same time.

● **Excessive alcohol consumption** – Excessive alcohol consumption can increase the risk of chronic diseases and conditions such as stroke, osteoporosis, and cancer [5]. By simply using moderation and restricting the number of alcoholic beverages during social activities, one can largely avoid this risk factor.

● **Smoking and Tobacco Use** – Any tobacco use, especially when excessive, can increase the risk of chronic diseases and conditions such as heart disease, stroke, type 2 diabetes, kidney disease, arthritis, cancer, and respiratory diseases [5]. The latest research has maintained that even secondhand smoke increases risk.

● **Exposure to environmental hazards** – Environmental hazards such as toxic chemicals, pollutants in the air and water, and harmful microorganisms can increase the risk of chronic disease even if the level of exposure is relatively low. Over time, such irritants can wear down our bodies.

● **Excessive sun exposure** – Some sun exposure can be healthy, but excessive sun exposure, specifically ultraviolet radiation, can increase our risk of skin cancer [7].

● **Lack of Sleep** – Insufficient sleep or poor sleep quality can increase the risk of chronic diseases such as diabetes and heart disease (cardiovascular disease) [8]. Lack of sleep can also contribute to other risk factors such as obesity and stress.

● **Excessive Stress** – Stress is largely ignored as a risk factor and is often cast aside as something we just have to live with. Unfortunately, a persistent high level of stress can increase the risk of a number of chronic diseases and health complications.

Introduction

*   *   *

The significance of knowing these risk factors is that it allows us to come up with a clear and concise roadmap to health and longevity. You may recognize that the risk factors are not some medical mystery or guarded secret. Most of us were probably aware of a number of them all along. However, in this era, it seems people need only a tiny bit of evidence to try something new, even irrelevant, so that they can ignore these risk factors. Unfortunately, they will find no panacea, and short-cutting will not work.

In any case, addressing these risk factors will enable us to focus on what is most important, rather than a random health goal that makes little difference in our lives. In fact, any good self-care system will contain common sense measures that are specifically designed to mitigate these risk factors.

*   *   *

Now, we move on to risk factors that **cannot be controlled or modified**. The good news is that the resulting impact of such risk factors can still be reduced. By addressing those risk factors that **can** be controlled, as stated previously, we may be able to turn off the triggers of related chronic diseases that are influenced by factors beyond our control.

The following are risk factors that we cannot control, but may still be able to mitigate indirectly.

● **Population subgroups** – Certain populations, which are based on demographics (such as race) and geographic area, can experience increased risk of some chronic diseases. For example, African American, Hispanic, and Native American subgroups have a greater risk of type 2 diabetes [9].

● **Gender** – Naturally, some chronic diseases are gender-dependent or carry a higher risk based on gender. An example is breast cancer. Although it does occur in men, it is more prevalent among females.

● **Age** – Age increases our risk of a wide range of chronic diseases, and, it may make other risk factors such as obesity and physical inactivity harder to contend with. As of yet, there is no obvious way to reverse the process; however, longevity can certainly be extended.

● **Genetic predisposition** – Our genes influence how susceptible we are to certain chronic diseases. For example, a family history of heart disease or certain cancers can indicate an existing genetic predisposition to those diseases. Genetic testing for certain at-risk genes can indicate higher risk levels and warrant medical screenings as a confirmation. Thankfully, we soon will all benefit from this technology.

*   *   *

It is important to address all of these risk factors in a timely manner. When it comes to chronic disease, everything adds up. And unfortunately, many risk factors can manifest themselves as diseases that elude detection until much later in life.

An emerging area of research called epigenetics focuses on how **<u>our lifestyle and environment can change the behavior of our genes</u>**. Recent studies have found that these changes can occur due to factors such as diet, exposure to pollutants, and even exercise [10]. If this phenomenon significantly influences susceptibility to chronic disease over time, we may be able to evolve, even during our lifespan in a sense, to possibly influence our long-term genetic fate. The promise of this research alone should make this a priority. So, if we start addressing these health issues early on, we will give even more time for our bodies to adapt sufficiently to new stimulus. Regardless of the outcome of such research though, any extra effort on our part will make us more resilient to chronic disease, no matter what the time frame is. Therefore, act now, for as we age, it will get harder to maintain positive control over our health.

A Common Sense Approach to Health and Longevity

The primary goal of this book is to provide a simple and easily-applied working system to improve health and increase lifespan. This book uses a multifaceted approach, while focusing on the most important risk factors in terms of chronic disease. It can, and should, be used by anyone, regardless of personal circumstance and state of health.

Of course, taking steps to improve health cannot be a one-time occurrence. It has to become part of a lifestyle or it will likely be diluted, even discontinued, at some point. Conventional wisdom dictates that great health benefits come from consistent, long-term action.

The focus of this book can be summarized into three main health imperatives.

● **Develop habits that strengthen the body over time** – A strong body will self-heal and will in turn strengthen our immune system and our internal cleansing processes. We will be able to cope with illnesses and environmental stressors more efficiently and effectively. Our muscles, bones, and joints will become stronger and more resilient to conditions that affect mobility and day-to-day functions. Together with advances in modern medicine, we will then be able to avoid many debilitating conditions that adversely affect quality of life and reduce lifespan. Note that it takes time for the body to adapt to stimuli and become stronger, so healthy habits must be established as early as possible.

● **Avoid unhealthy extremes** – Extremes, or abnormal or excessive behaviors, can get us into trouble when it comes to long-term health. Certain bad habits, such as smoking and excessive alcohol consumption, can cause irreversible damage and catch up with us later in life. Although this is obvious to the average person, there are more subtle ways to experience an unhealthy extreme. Eating too much of one type of food, not getting enough sleep, and sitting for too long are examples of behavior that can discreetly and adversely impact health over time. We can and should avoid such extremes and learn to practice moderation in our daily lives.

● **Minimize unnecessary exposure to environmental hazards** – Examples of environmental hazards include ultraviolet radiation, pollutants, toxic chemicals, allergens, harmful microorganisms, and strong electromagnetic fields.   Many of us live in crowded, urban, high-tech environments, surrounded by such hazards on a daily basis. Trying to quantify long-term exposure can seem like a daunting task, since such hazards may not seem like much of a threat at first. However, there is danger when we do not take into account that the exposure, which can last over decades or even an entire lifespan, has the potential to create some level of internal damage. Accumulated damage can have a big impact later in life and take us by surprise in the form of illness and disease.

How This Book is organized

With this introduction, the need for a comprehensive system for long-term health is clear. Naturally, we need to focus on a suitable range of risk factors so we can act immediately to prevent the onset of chronic diseases most likely to impact our lives. It is not enough to focus on just one. If we do that, we risk entering a phase of life that looks a lot like the vicious circle illustrated in figure 2.

This book covers a broad range of topics. You will notice some of these topics are somewhat unconventional for a book about health. This does not make them any less valid. They are intentionally included as a way to inform and motivate ourselves to look at common health problems from multiple angles.

These are the topics that will be addressed in the remainder of this book.

Chapter 1: Diet and Nutrition – This chapter specifies the components of a healthy diet, along with recommendations for preventing unhealthy weight gain. It covers alternative sources of nutrition, but stresses eating whole foods as the primary source of nutrients instead of relying on supplements.

Introduction

Chapter 2: At the Grocery Store – Since nutrition is so important to health, it is important to know how to shop for the best food. At the very least, one must know how to read and evaluate food product labels. One should also understand how hidden ingredients, such as food additives, affect the nutritional quality of food and impact health.

Chapter 3: Kitchen Basics – Most probably do not know how food preparation influences health and nutrition. Processing, preservation, and cooking can all impact the quality and safety of food as well as its nutritional value.

Chapter 4: Exercise and Physical Activity – Inactivity is a major risk factor for chronic disease. This chapter covers how aerobic activity, strength training, and other physical activities should be incorporated into a weekly schedule for maximum benefit.

Chapter 5: Sleep and Stress Management – This chapter discusses how to get the optimal amount of sleep, which is vital to long-term health. In addition to a lack of sleep, excessive stress is a harmful condition that is often overlooked. Since both conditions are interrelated, various methods for coping with stress are also covered.

Chapter 6: Environmental Chemical Hazards – Sources of toxic chemicals exist all around us. And exposure to household chemicals, building materials, and air pollution can adversely impact health. Reducing exposure to these types of chemicals and others will be discussed.

Chapter 7: Biological Pollutants and Germs – We share the same space with numerous tiny organisms and substances, both inside and outside the home. In high concentrations, many of them can cause illness. This chapter provides information on how to minimize exposure to such irritants, including allergens and germs.

Chapter 8: Technology Related Health Hazards – The threat from long-term exposure to electromagnetic fields is not well-known. The dangers of such radiation will be discussed along with other common health problems associated with modern technology.

Chapter 9: Cosmetics and Skin Protection – Cosmetic products contain certain substances that can be absorbed by layers of the skin and end up in the bloodstream. This chapter will cover how to minimize exposure to such substances, as well as how to prevent excessive sun exposure, which can increase the risk of skin cancer.

Conclusion – This section discusses some general recommendations on health, alternative treatments, and the nature of medical and scientific research.

*   *   *

Note that this book is not an encyclopedia on health and longevity. It is also not an academic textbook. The concepts are not complicated and therefore should actually be intuitive to the average reader. At the same time, the science behind many of these concepts, although sophisticated, is convincing enough to encourage anyone to effect real improvements in their health. In this regard, we will follow the consensus of scientific research, instead of a single sensationalized study or observation.

Also, you will notice that this book combines a number of seemingly disparate, yet related concepts. Some will come from conventional knowledge about health and longevity. Others will be fashioned from information that is typically not well-known, but very important from the standpoint of health.

This book is unique in that it consolidates approaches to health in a world with an endless amount of data that is often conflicting and confusing. This book is also meant to help you think about health a little differently, but in a way that should be somewhat innate, like a dose of common sense. You probably suspected the truth to some of this information all along, but wondered why so little of it is discussed in the mainstream.

Introduction

It is important to note that every person is different in terms of genetic makeup, susceptibility to disease, environment, individual needs, and stage in life. So, many of the guidelines presented will apply to a broader audience rather than a particular group.

Note that this information is not a substitute for medical advice. The purpose of the book is to help you mitigate the risk factors of chronic disease and stay out the hospital emergency room. Its focus is on long-term health and it addresses topics that are usually outside the scope of most books on the market. If you suspect you have a health problem, it is not the time to shun traditional medical treatment or advice. In fact, most of what is covered in this book will probably compliment whatever your doctor recommends and help get you back on track.

We now proceed to what is perhaps the most important area of health, our diet.

Chapter 1: Diet and Nutrition

The Importance of Diet and Nutrition

The importance of diet in overall health is often considered common knowledge. However, both diet and nutrition continue to present a global health challenge. Despite the abundance of research and information available to the public, factors such as obesity and poor nutrition continue to play a significant role in the pervasiveness of chronic disease. Many of these diseases are preventable or can at least be mitigated with proper diet alone.

Consider the following **health problems** that are implicated by **poor diet and inadequate nutrition** [11].

● **Heart disease** is influenced by factors such as **high cholesterol**, **high blood pressure**, **diabetes**, and **unhealthy weight gain**. All of these conditions are influenced heavily by diet and nutrition.

● **High blood pressure** is a condition that has been linked to **heart disease**, **stroke**, and **kidney disease**. It is increased by factors such as **unhealthy weight gain**, **heavy sodium consumption**, and **insufficient potassium**, to name a few.

● **Cancer** has also been associated with improper diet. Included are breast, uterine, colon, kidney, and esophagus cancers.

● **Diabetes** is a metabolic disorder that is heavily influenced by diet. **Overweight and obese individuals** have a higher risk of developing diabetes.

● **Osteoporosis** results from a **loss of bone mass and density**. Adequate nutrition and exercise are required to maintain sufficient bone mass to reduce the **risk of injury and disability** from accidents.

*　　*　　*

This list is far from complete but it does highlight some of the significant diseases that diet plays a role in. And you'll notice also that diet is a prime factor, directly or indirectly, within the vicious circle of chronic disease (see Introduction, figure 2). The good news is that we have the power to mitigate these conditions without drugs or other medical interventions.

Consuming a healthy diet is one of the most significant things we can do to increase lifespan and live a healthy life. It is amazing that something as simple as eating a nutritious well-balanced diet can have such a profound effect on one's health. In fact, organizations such as the American Heart Association, Centers for Disease Control, Department of Health and Human Services, National Institutes of Health, World Health Organization, and many others all echo the importance of a healthy diet in managing disease. The importance of diet cannot be understated.

What Makes a Healthy Diet?

The primary goals of a diet are essentially to **maintain a healthy weight** and **acquire enough nutrients to support an active and healthy lifestyle**. Developing an optimal diet is often easier said than done. The problem is not so much in getting information on diet and nutrition as it is in filtering out what is useful and what isn't. It can be a daunting task without a background in nutrition or some other appropriate expertise. Numerous diet advertisements, health bulletins, news stories, online blogs, and other sources claim to have the answers on what we should and should not be eating. It is easy to become disenchanted and just forget about the whole diet thing altogether. Luckily, all of the work has been done for us. The latest information has already been compiled and studied. Consensus has been, for the most part, achieved in reference to what is really important about diet and nutrition. We just need to know where to look.

There are already well-established sets of dietary guidelines that are easy to follow and recommended by experts in the field. They don't have fancy rules or point systems, and are easy to incorporate into almost any lifestyle. By simply following the forthcoming guidelines, you can be sure you are satisfying nutritional requirements for optimal health and thus stave off the most common causes of disease and disability.

In general, to obtain all the nutrients you need to prevent chronic disease, you need to eat a variety of nutrient-dense foods in all food groups. These foods contain vitamins, minerals, and other nutrients that are important to maintain good health. It is broadly agreed that this can be accomplished by incorporating the following into your diet [11].

● Eat more **fruits and vegetables**. Include a **variety of different types** of vegetables including dark green, red and orange vegetables, and beans and peas. This will ensure you get an adequate amount of vitamins and minerals in your diet.

● Eat more **whole grains**. Whole grains are unrefined, which means the entire grain seed is used, and the germ and bran have not been removed during processing. Use whole grains to replace refined grains, such as white flour, white rice, and white bread, whenever possible. This will give you energy and ensure you get plenty of fiber in your diet.

● Choose **non-fat or low-fat dairy products**.

● Eat a variety of **healthy protein foods** such as fish, poultry, eggs, beans and peas, and nuts. This will ensure you get enough protein in your diet.

● Limit red meat and sugary food and drinks.

*   *   *

In particular, fruits and vegetables have the highest value in terms of overall nutrient density and should be consumed in the greatest quantities [12]. However, by eating foods from all of these groups, you greatly decrease risk of nutrient deficiency, and thus substantially reduce the risk of chronic disease over the course of one's life.

If you do nothing else but follow these general rules, you will be well on your way toward accomplishing your long-term health goals.

Diet Plans for Health

There are a number of different formalized diet plans and recommendations that can be considered optimal for preventing chronic disease. Some of the options include the USDA My Plate, Harvard Healthy Eating Plate, TLC, DASH, Mediterranean, and Mayo Clinic diets, among others. Choosing any one of these plans would satisfy nutritional requirements.

Additionally, some of these plans are tweaked to address a specific chronic disease or condition. For example, the DASH diet plan (Dietary Approaches to Stop Hypertension) is designed to help lower blood pressure [13]. The TLC diet plan (Therapeutic Lifestyle Changes Diet) is recommended by the National Institutes of Health to lower cholesterol and reduce risk of heart disease [14]. The Mediterranean diet is inspired by studies showing that people in Mediterranean countries who eat certain foods have a lower risk of heart disease in general [15].

The advantage of following such diet plans is that they give more specific recommendations to help you make the right day-to-day food choices. The Harvard Healthy Eating Plate, for example, is good for health, and is flexible and easy to follow [16]. Here are some of the specifics.

- **Vegetables and fruit (50%)** – Approximately **half of each plate** should consist of vegetables and fruit. Conventional vegetables and fruit sold at a grocery store should suffice. Try to include a variety. Potatoes and potato fries are not considered part of this group.

- **Whole grains (25%)** – Approximately **one quarter of each plate** should consist of whole grain foods. This includes whole grain breads (e.g. whole grain sliced bread, bagels, muffins, rolls, pitas, and tortillas), whole grain cereals (e.g. oats, barley, buckwheat, and shredded wheat), brown rice, and whole wheat pastas. Refined grains such as white rice, pasta, and bread, along with potatoes and potato fries, should be very limited.

● **Healthy Protein (25%)** – Approximately <u>**one quarter of each plate**</u> should consist of lean proteins such as chicken and fish and other healthy protein sources such as beans, nuts, and tofu. Red meats, including steak and ground meat, should be limited. Processed meats, including bacon, sausage, bologna, and salami, should be largely avoided.

● **Water, coffee, and tea** – Drinks can include water, coffee, and tea. Sugary drinks such as soda, energy drinks, and sport drinks should be avoided. A small glass of fruit juice each day is acceptable.

● **Healthy Oils** – Oils such as olive, canola, coconut, soy, corn, sesame, peanut, flaxseed, and other vegetable oils should be <u>**consumed in moderation**</u>. Use of butter should be very limited.

● **Milk and dairy** – Milk and dairy products such as cheese, yogurt, and sour cream should be reduced to about <u>**one or two servings each day**</u>. It is interesting to note that consuming too much of these products can result in overconsumption of certain nutrients such as saturated fat.

*   *   *

So, eating healthy does not have to be a complicated process. It is also not necessary to review every diet plan in existence to find the magic formula. Just choose a reputable diet plan that is easiest to follow. Specifically, it should be the one you are most likely to stick with over the long term. Or, you can just follow the basic dietary guidelines outlined earlier. This will ensure you are consuming the nutrients you need to avoid nutritional deficiencies and help prevent the worst of the chronic diseases. A healthy diet really is common sense.

General Recommendations for Weight Loss

Obesity is known to be a major risk factor for a host of chronic diseases. Furthermore, when it comes to obesity, what you eat is probably the most significant causal factor. So, it goes without saying that tailoring a diet to maintain a healthy weight is paramount. The **formula for weight loss** is actually quite simple. When accomplished through diet, weight loss can be achieved by **reducing the number of calories** you eat so that you are eating fewer calories than your body is expending through physical activity [17]. However, there is more to it than that. A study from Harvard University concluded that the quality of calories consumed may be more important than the actual number [18]. For example, processed foods such as white bread, white rice, and some breakfast cereals can have an adverse effect on blood sugar and hamper weight loss efforts even as fewer calories are consumed. That means that we should be **consuming more quality foods** (e.g. more fruits and vegetables, whole grains, and lean protein) as well as cutting calories.

In addition, there are a number of dietary shortcuts we may be able to use to make losing weight easier and help accelerate the process. Consider the following general recommendations.

• **Eat a healthy diet** – This is the simplest action you can take. By following the general guidelines for a healthy diet as previously discussed, you are consuming quality calories instead of empty ones that contribute to weight gain. To help with choosing the right foods, follow a particular healthy diet plan such as the TLC, DASH, or Mediterranean diet, or refer to the Harvard Healthy Eating Plate recommendations. Doing so, even without a specialized weight loss plan, will help you lose weight and keep it off for good.

• **Follow a specialized weight loss diet plan** – A number of specialized diet systems and guidelines are available to help lose weight. Some of them are advertised specifically for that purpose. Choosing the right plan can be an overwhelming task with so many available, especially if you don't have someone you trust nudging you in the right direction. To give you a general idea on just how many of these diets are out there, the U.S. News and World Report compiled a list of diets in 2015 (table 2) and ranked them according to different health criteria [19]. The top-ranked diets for weight loss are marked with a circle.

Abs Diet		Glycemic-Index Diet		South Beach Diet	
Acid Alkaline Diet		HMR Diet	● ■	Spark Solution Diet	
Anti-Inflammatory Diet		Jenny Craig	● ■	Supercharged Hormone Diet	
Atkins	●	Macrobiotic Diet		The Fast Diet	
Biggest Loser Diet	●	Mayo Clinic Diet		TLC Diet	
Body Reset Diet		Medifast	■	Traditional Asian Diet	
DASH Diet		Mediterranean Diet		Vegan Diet	●
Dukan Diet		Nutrisystem	■	Vegetarian Diet	
Eco-Atkins Diet		Ornish Diet		Volumetrics	●
Engine 2 Diet		Paleo Diet		Weight Watchers	● ■
Flat Belly Diet		Raw Food Diet	●	Zone Diet	
Flexitarian Diet	●	Slim-Fast	● ■		

Table 2 – List of popular diets. Diets marked with a circle are ranked as the top diets for overall __weight loss__ according to U.S. News and World Report. Diets marked with a square have commercial food products associated with the diet (costs vary). These commercial products will help manage portions for you and can make it easier to commit to a program.

Some of these diets have commercial food products that are part of the diet plan. They cost money, but in return they provide the convenience of not having to plan, measure portions, or prepare meals every day. It is important to point out that, with any plan, there will be separate grocery expenses. In some cases, you may have to buy reading materials and recipe books to better understand the diet in question.

The important part of choosing a weight loss diet is to find the one that works for you. Each person has unique circumstances that may make one diet preferable over another. You will also find that many of these plans recommend a regular exercise regimen as well to speed up the process. In any case, if the diet is healthy and you can stay with the program until you achieve significant weight loss, then that diet is the best one for you, regardless of any ranking.

● **Drink more water** – Replace high-calorie sugary drinks such as soft drinks, fruit juices, specialty coffee drinks, energy drinks, and sport drinks with water throughout the day and during meals [20]. This will cut a significant number of calories from your diet. In addition, drinking extra water before a meal and during a meal may achieve a feeling of fullness.

● **Eat filling foods** – Filling foods generally contain more fiber, protein, and water [21]. The best filling foods, however, are the low-calorie options such as fruit and vegetables. Other options include baked potatoes, oatmeal, whole grains, air-popped popcorn, lean protein foods, eggs, beans and lentils, and soups, which contain lots of extra water. So, as explained earlier, fill more of the plate with these types of foods, and reduce portion sizes of the others.

● **Limit intake of high-calorie processed food** – Some examples of high-calorie processed foods include fried foods, fatty milk products, crackers, cookies, chips, sugary foods, and fatty meats such as bologna, bacon, and sausages. By reducing the amount of these foods on your plate, you will drastically reduce the calorie count and eat healthier in the process.

● **Reduce portion sizes** – Sometimes it is difficult to determine portion sizes. Initially, you may have to measure portions carefully when preparing meals at home. After a few times, however, you should be able to eyeball it. For example, one serving of meat or poultry is about the size of a deck of cards. When you are not preparing your own meals, you can always cut down the portions by ordering small size meals or choosing appetizers in lieu of a high-calorie entrée. You can also save the second half of a large meal so you can enjoy it again later. If you have the discipline, portion control is a good way to enjoy certain types of food without overdoing it. Some of the weight loss diets, such as Medifast and Nutrisystem, control these portions meticulously for you.

● **Eat textured foods that promote chewing** – Foods that are tougher to chew or require more attentive eating will help slow you down and reduce the amount of food consumed over time. In addition to feeling full, more chewing will improve digestion. Try this approach on all foods you consume as well.

● **Practice intermittent fasting** – Fasting is not the same as starving. With fasting, you just choose to limit calorie intake by restricting consumption of food for pre-determined periods of time [22]. The objective is not nutritional deficiency, but simply a reduction of the daily caloric intake to a safe but effective level to promote weight loss or other health benefits. It may involve skipping a meal, but it doesn't have to be this way. Fasting cycles can be short (e.g. skipping a single meal) or long (e.g. up to 24 hours). Choosing long cycles may not be necessary, but some research suggests there may be some additional health benefits. Until we know for sure what is safe and effective, shorter cycles are probably advisable.

Fasting is not for everyone. For some individuals, it may lead to overeating due to a more intense feeling of hunger. If, however, it works for you and fits your lifestyle, it may help to reduce overall calorie intake. It is a good idea to check with a health professional before embarking on more extreme fasting schedules, as fasting incorrectly could lead to nutritional deficiencies and could be harmful.

Alternative Sources of Nutrition

Many people would like to go the extra mile to ensure they are getting optimal nutrition. This typically involves using some form of dietary supplement containing vitamins, minerals, and herbs. If the size of the supplement industry is any indication, the use of supplements is widespread and growing. Supplements are attractive in that they promise a shortcut to nutrition when one is following a largely unhealthy diet. Some also believe that supplements confer some additional health benefits beyond that of a normal diet. Unfortunately, scientific research has shown that the benefits of such alternative sources of nutrition are limited and are not nearly as impressive as the advertisements would have you believe. Even widely used supplements, such as multivitamins, lack the consensus to support a recommendation for or against their use in preventing disease or increasing longevity.

Conventional wisdom has shown that most **nutrition should come from whole foods first, then fortified foods, and last from supplements** [23]. Eating whole foods is the best way to get all the nutrients you ever need. Priority should be given to the more nutrient-dense foods, such as fruits and vegetables. Fortified foods (foods with artificially-added nutrients) and supplements may be appropriate in specific situations when certain whole foods are not available.

Fortified foods are foods that have one or more nutrients added to them through the manufacturing process. Examples include cereals fortified with fiber, and eggs enriched with omega-3 fatty acids. Fortified foods are still preferable to supplements since nutrients consumed in this way will be stored more efficiently and effectively than supplements taken intermittently. However, these foods are still considered inferior to whole foods.

Dietary supplements on the other hand come in many forms including tablets, capsules, soft gels, chewable forms, gum candies, liquids, and powders. They can be used to treat certain nutritional deficiencies, but their effectiveness in preventing disease is questionable and has been a debate issue for some time.

It may come as a surprise that **supplements are intended to be used as a last resort and are rarely needed by healthy individuals**.

With respect to supplements, a poor diet will still largely negate any benefits you may receive by consuming them. Consider also that whole foods contain other potentially important ingredients that are typically left out of supplements, such as phytonutrients. Phytonutrients are chemicals in plants that may provide additional health benefits when consumed. Still, it is not unusual to find people who have justified the need to try new supplements or consume extra nutrients, just in case.

It is also important to note that there are some situations in which taking supplements are absolutely justified. For example, they can be used to help treat a known nutritional deficiency or when recommended by a doctor to treat an illness. They can also be used by certain groups of people that have a special need (e.g. prenatal vitamins for pregnant women or vitamin D for older adults). However, in most other cases, the justification is lacking in terms of scientific evidence.

Consider the following disadvantages of supplements before relying on them too heavily to satisfy perceived nutritional needs.

• **Poor bioavailability when compared to food** – Bioavailability is a term used to describe the absorption and utilization of a nutrient in the body. Often, very little of a supplement is absorbed by the body. This is why the dosage is often so high. On top of that, there are questions as to whether the known mechanism of action for a nutrient in the body is the same when taken in excess or taken in a form other than whole food.

• **Difficulty in determining proper dosage** – The human body is complex and every person is different, so the exact dosage needed to be effective is hard to determine. This may explain why there are so many variations in dosage for supplements on the market. With these variations, there is also a risk of taking too much of a nutrient. Between whole foods and fortified foods, most of us are already getting enough nutrients. Since many of us take supplements throughout the day, at some point, the increased dosages may actually become hazardous to health.

● **Interactions with other nutrients** – Some nutrients require other nutrients to be effective. Food already contains an ideal mixture of different nutrients and compounds, which allow for better utilization. Attempting to do the same with a complex combination of different supplements is very difficult, if not impossible.

● **Creation of imbalances in the body** – Taking too much of a supplement can create a systemic imbalance. This imbalance can possibly cause damage and become hazardous to long-term health. For example, some studies suggest that taking high doses of antioxidants, such a vitamin C and E, could shut down some of the self-repair mechanisms in the body normally stimulated by elements called free radicals [24]. We may take supplements to get rid of these free radicals, unaware that we actually need them to function properly.

● **Possible increase in disease risk** – This is the opposite of what we want to accomplish with proper nutrition. While we are taking supplements to prevent chronic disease and improve health, it is possible that we are, instead, increasing our risk of chronic disease. For example, some studies have suggested that popular supplements such as beta-carotene, selenium, and folic acid can increase the risk of cancer when taken in excess [25].

● **Possible interactions with medication** – Although supplements are unlikely to provide a desired benefit for health, they may in fact interfere with important medical treatments by interacting negatively with medications. Supplements can also interfere with over-the-counter drugs. To reduce this risk, you should probably check with your healthcare provider about supplements you are taking, especially if medication is prescribed.

- **Unknown ingredients** – Supplements are not regulated like drugs. The Food and Drug Administration does not fully investigate supplements before they are put on the market [26]. As a result, you may be consuming harmful byproducts or other hidden ingredients along with the nutrient.

- **Unknown long-term side effects** – Although most supplements are deemed safe for intermittent use, long-term side effects in many cases are not well known. Most studies deal with high dosages or shorter time spans. But, with newer supplements, it is often not possible to ascertain what all the effects will be over the course of a lifespan or many years of use.

- **Additional expense** – In addition to groceries, spending money on supplements can be expensive. Consider that supplements containing water-soluble vitamins, such as vitamin C and B-complex, are not retained in the body and therefore have to be taken more often and in greater quantities. As a result, Americans continue to spend billions of extra dollars each year on such supplements.

*   *   *

The bottom line is: until we know more about these supplements and can prove that they provide additional protection from chronic disease, we should not rely on them as a primary source of nutrition. Therefore, since supplements will not likely confer any benefits beyond what you get from a healthy diet, whole foods remain clearly superior for avoiding nutritional deficiencies.

Dietary Sources of Nutrients

If you still feel the need to increase certain vitamins and minerals as supplements in your diet, know that there are available alternatives. For instance, consider consuming more of the certain foods that contain those nutrients.

Table 3 lists essential nutrients that have a role in reducing the risk of chronic disease [27, 28, 29]. The top dietary sources for each of those nutrients are also included.

When talking about reducing risks, the nutrients themselves don't have magical properties when consumed in excess. The real benefit is conferred only by consuming an adequate amount necessary to **avoid nutritional deficiencies that lead to chronic disease**. Remember that you only need enough of an essential nutrient to stay healthy. Consuming more than you need is just not necessary.

There are many supplements on the market that claim to have additional health benefits. There are also studies published, almost daily, touting the next magical cure or key to longevity. Most of these claims, however, are simply a matter of wishful thinking. It is important to note that science is an ongoing process and consensus takes time when it comes to determining whether benefits are real and measurable. In most cases the benefits are exaggerated. Often a study will show that supplementation works really well for mice. Unfortunately, those results do not necessarily translate well to humans. What is painfully obvious is that the general population is often easily diverted by unsubstantiated promises of well-being. In many cases, the only positive effect from supplements comes from a strong belief in a healthy response. Like a placebo, other variables enter the equation, but the results, if any, do not support the supplement as a critical factor in what is a perceived health benefit.

Nutrient	Top Dietary Sources
Biotin (Vitamin H)	Brewer's yeast; cooked eggs, egg yolks; sardines; nuts (e.g. almonds, peanuts, pecans, walnuts), nut butters; soybeans; legumes (e.g. beans, black-eyed peas); whole grains; cauliflower; bananas; mushrooms
Calcium	Cheese (e.g. parmesan, Romano, gruyere, cheddar, American, mozzarella, feta); milk; yogurt; tofu, blackstrap molasses; almonds; brewer's yeast; bok choy; Brazil nuts; broccoli; cabbage; dried figs; kelp; dark leafy green vegetables (e.g. turnip, collard, mustard greens, kale, Swiss chard); hazelnuts; oysters; canned sardines, salmon; fortified foods (e.g. breakfast cereals, juices, rice milk, soy milk, tofu)
Dietary Fiber	Fruits and vegetables; whole grains; wheat and corn bran; dried beans and peas
Folate or Folic Acid (Vitamin B9)	Dark leafy green vegetables (e.g. spinach, turnip, beets, mustard greens), asparagus, Brussel sprouts; lima beans; soybeans; beef liver; brewer's yeast; root vegetables (e.g. carrots, radishes); whole grains; wheat germ; bulgur wheat; kidney beans; white beans; lima beans; salmon; orange juice; avocado; milk; fortified foods (e.g. breakfast cereals)
Iodine	Iodized salt; shellfish (e.g. crab, lobster, clams, shrimp, oysters) ; white deep water fish (e.g. cod, tuna); brown seaweed kelp; garlic; lima beans; sesame seeds; soybeans; spinach; Swiss chard; summer squash; turnip greens
Iron	Organ meats (e.g. liver); lean red meat (e.g. lean steak, beef, and pork); poultry (e.g. chicken, turkey); fish; shellfish (e.g. oysters); dried beans and peas; legumes (e.g. beans, lentils, peas); nuts; seeds; whole grains; dark molasses; green leafy vegetables; fortified foods (e.g. breakfast cereals)
Magnesium	Tofu; legumes; whole grains; green leafy vegetables; wheat bran; Brazil nuts; soybean flour; almonds; cashews; blackstrap molasses; pumpkin and squash seeds; pine nuts; black walnuts; peanuts; whole wheat flour; oat flour; beet greens; spinach; pistachio nuts; shredded wheat; bran cereals; oatmeal; bananas; baked potatoes; chocolate; cocoa powder; herbs; spices

(Table 3 continued)

Nutrient	Top Dietary Sources
Niacin (Vitamin B3)	Beets; brewer's yeast; beef liver; beef kidney; fish; salmon; swordfish; tuna; sunflower seeds; peanuts; fortified foods (e.g. breads, cereals)
Pantothenic Acid (Vitamin B5)	Brewer's yeast; corn; cauliflower; kale; broccoli; tomatoes; avocado; legumes (e.g. lentils); egg yolks; beef; organ meats; poultry; milk; split peas; peanuts; soybeans; sweet potatoes; sunflower seeds; whole grains; lobster; wheat germ; salmon
Potassium	Bananas; citrus juices (e.g. orange, lemon, grapefruit); avocados; cantaloupes; tomatoes; potatoes; lima beans; flounder; salmon; cod; chicken
Protein	Meats; poultry; fish; eggs; dairy products (e.g. milk, yogurt, cheese); soy; beans; legumes; nuts; nut butters; wheat germ
Riboflavin (Vitamin B2)	Brewer's yeast; almonds; organ meats; whole grains; wheat germ; wild rice; mushrooms; soybeans; milk; yogurt; eggs; broccoli; Brussels sprouts; spinach; fortified foods (e.g. flours, cereals)
Selenium	Brewer's yeast; wheat germ; liver; butter; fish (e.g. mackerel, tuna, halibut, flounder, herring, smelt); shellfish (e.g. oysters, scallops, lobster); garlic; whole grains; sunflower seeds; Brazil nuts
Thiamine (Vitamin B1)	Pork; organ meats; whole-grains; legumes; wheat germ; bran; brewer's yeast; blackstrap molasses
Vitamin A (Retinol)	Beef; eggs; dairy products (e.g. milk, yogurt, butter, cottage cheese, cheese)
Vitamin B12	Fish; shellfish; dairy products; organ meats (e.g. liver, kidney) eggs; beef; pork
Vitamin B6	Chicken; turkey; tuna; salmon; shrimp; milk; cheese; lentils; beans; spinach; carrots; brown rice; bran; sunflower seeds; wheat germ; whole-grain flour
Vitamin C	Oranges; watermelon; papaya; grapefruit; cantaloupe; strawberries; kiwifruit; mango; broccoli; tomatoes; Brussel sprouts; cauliflower; cabbage; leafy greens (e.g. turnips, spinach); red and green peppers; tomatoes; potatoes; winter squash; raspberries; blueberries; cranberries; pineapple; fortified foods (e.g. juices, beverages)

(Table 3 continued)

Nutrient	Top Dietary Sources
Vitamin D	Fatty fish (e.g. salmon, mackerel, tuna, sardines, herring); fortified foods (e.g. milk, cereals); eggs
Vitamin E	Wheat germ; liver; eggs; nuts (e.g. almonds, hazelnuts, walnuts); sunflower seeds; corn-oil margarine; mayonnaise; vegetable oils; dark leafy green vegetables (e.g. spinach, turnip, beets, collard, mustard greens, kale); sweet potatoes; avocado; asparagus; yams
Vitamin K	Beef liver; green tea; turnip greens; broccoli; kale; spinach; cabbage; asparagus; dark green lettuce
Zinc	Oysters; red meat; poultry; cheese (e.g. ricotta; Swiss; gouda); shellfish (e.g. shrimp, crab); legumes (e.g. lima beans, black-eyed peas, pinto beans, soybeans, peanuts); whole grains; miso; tofu; brewer's yeast; cooked greens; mushrooms; green beans; tahini; pumpkin; sunflower seeds

Table 3 – List of essential nutrients that are both important to health and that have a role in reducing the risk of chronic disease. The top dietary sources have a relatively high concentration of the nutrients indicated.

Often times, the nutrients provided by these special supplements have an alternative food source. In these cases, it would be much safer to consume the additional nutrients from a food source rather than experiment with the potentially high dosage of a dietary supplement. For some nutrients, however, there is no food substitute. Sometimes we produce the compound or nutrient in our bodies naturally. At other times, the nutrient is unnatural and is simply not needed. In this case, the supplement is meant to act more like a drug, except that it doesn't face the same level of scrutiny as drugs do by regulatory agencies. This is why one might want to think long and hard before taking such supplements. It is advisable at least to wait until more definitive evidence is made available confirming their benefits and their safety after long-term usage. Alternatively, you should ask your doctor how safe they are.

Table 4 lists some popular supplements and their alternative food sources (if any) [29]. Possible uses are also included to illustrate some of the potential health benefits [30]. The benefits are only included in this table if the supplement is deemed **effective** or **likely effective** based on methodology from the National Medicines Comprehensive Database [31]. To fit the criteria, they must pass a very high standard based on reliable evidence. According to the same standard, any other use is not supported by sufficient evidence for a particular disease or condition. In this case, more research is probably needed before experimenting with the supplement. There are better and more reliable alternatives.

Supplement	Possible Uses	Top Dietary Sources
5-Hydroxytryptophan (or 5-HTP)	Not applicable	No significant dietary sources
Alpha-lipoic Acid	Not applicable	Red meat (e.g. roast, beef, hamburger, pork); organ meat (e.g. liver); yeast (e.g. brewer's yeast)
Beta-carotene	Reduce sun sensitivity for people with certain conditions	Yellow, orange, and green leafy vegetables (e.g. carrots, spinach, lettuce, tomatoes, sweet potatoes, broccoli, winter squash); cantaloupe
Carnitine	Not applicable	No significant dietary sources
Chondroitin	Not applicable	No significant dietary sources
Coenzyme Q10 (or CoQ-10)	Treat Coenzyme Q10 deficiency	Oily fish (e.g. salmon, tuna); organ meats (e.g. liver); whole grains
Colloidal Silver	Not applicable	No significant dietary sources
Creatine	Not applicable	Wild game meats (e.g. elk, rabbit, venison, duck); red meat (e.g. lean steak, beef, pork); fish (e.g. herring, salmon, tuna)

(Table 4 continued)

Supplement	Possible Uses	Top Dietary Sources
DHEA	Not applicable	No significant dietary sources
Fish Oil (Omega-3 fatty acids)	Reduce triglyceride level	Enhanced foods (e.g. eggs); fish (e.g. salmon, mackerel, halibut, sardines, tuna, herring); oils (e.g. flaxseed, canola, soybean); pumpkin seeds; purslane; walnuts
Glucosamine Sulfate	Reduce osteoarthritis symptoms in some people	No significant dietary sources
Melatonin	Treat some sleep disorders in some people	No significant dietary sources
Probiotics and prebiotics (e.g. Lactobacillus acidophilus	Not applicable	Enriched foods (e.g. milk); yogurt; onions; tomatoes; bananas; honey; barley; garlic; wheat
S-Adenosylmethionine (or SAMe)	Reduce depression symptoms, reduce osteoarthritis symptoms	No significant dietary sources
Sulfur (e.g. MSM, DMSO)	Not applicable	Eggs; meat; poultry; fish; legumes; garlic; onions; Brussel sprouts; asparagus; kale; wheat germ
Turmeric and Curcumin	Not applicable	Seasonings (e.g. curry powders)

Table 4 – List of popular supplements. Possible uses are included if supplementation is deemed effective or likely effective based on available evidence. Top dietary sources have a relatively high concentration of the particular nutrient.

Herbal Supplements

The use of plants or herbs for healing has been around for a very long time. They have been used to treat or relieve symptoms of all sorts of illnesses from the common cold to healing of wounds and cuts. Table 5 lists some of the common herbal supplements.

Aloe	Flaxseed	Lavender
Chamomile	Garlic	Lemon balm
Cranberry	Ginger	St. John's Wort
Devil's Claw	Ginkgo	Tea tree
Echinacea	Ginseng	Valerian
Eucalyptus	Green Tea	

Table 5 – Common Herbal Supplements. The use of such supplements for prevention or treatment of chronic diseases is largely unsubstantiated.

As a medicine or supplement, there are many ways to consume herbs. They can be made into teas, tinctures, infusions, ointments, oils, syrups, poultices, or powders.

Make no mistake; some of these herbs are potent when taken in high doses. Because of this, there is a chance they can cause health problems if utilized incorrectly. No doubt they may also interfere with certain medications.

Unfortunately, despite the fact that they can initiate such reactions in the short-term, the evidence supporting any sort of long-term benefit is unsubstantiated. Some people would like to believe that an herb or plant supplement is a panacea for disease in general. However, this is completely unrealistic. Aside from St. John's Wort to help treat mild depression in some people, there is little definitive proof supporting the use of such supplements, in any form, for the prevention or treatment of any chronic disease [30].

Another part of the problem is that the effectiveness of an herb or plant is greatly influenced by the individual consuming it, the type of plant, the preparation, and even the soil it is grown in. The variables that determine the effectiveness are varied and unpredictable. That is part of the reason why taking them is often hit-or-miss for even minor ailments. That is not to say that herbal medicine is irrelevant in helping to treat the symptoms of some acute illness or injury. However, as for management of more serious diseases or chronic conditions, they are probably not a permanent or reliable substitute for modern medicine. As far as prevention is concerned, there are better alternatives out there. Lately, herbal supplements are being investigated more thoroughly for long-term health benefits, and that is expected to continue for some time. For now, though, it would be best to wait for more evidence.

Putting it All Together

The importance of diet and nutrition in preventing chronic disease is well-known. As previously discussed, following a healthy diet should not be a complicated endeavor. By consuming more nutrient-dense foods such as fruits and vegetables, we can maintain a healthy weight and reduce the risk of nutritional deficiencies that contribute to chronic disease and disability. This is, perhaps, the most important thing we can do to improve long-term health.

If you feel you cannot satisfy all your nutritional requirements through food, supplements are unlikely to help much, if at all. Remember, in most cases, the evidence is simply insufficient to justify reliance on supplements for nutrition or any health claim that goes beyond what a normal diet would accomplish. Unless you have a medical condition that necessitates alternative sources of nutrition, making minor adjustments to your diet is a far more effective, and convenient, measure for reducing chronic disease risk.

To help you establish new patterns of behavior, a summary of important action steps are included at the end of each chapter, starting with this one. Try to incorporate them into your life as soon as possible. Remember that your body needs time to adapt to new stimuli, so starting early and staying consistent is key to long-term health.

The following action steps can be taken right away.

ACTION STEPS

1.	To <u>maintain healthy weight</u> and <u>acquire enough nutrients</u>, consume nutrient-dense foods in all food groups. This includes <u>fruits and vegetables</u>, <u>whole grains</u>, <u>low-fat dairy products</u>, and <u>lean protein foods</u>.
2.	For <u>weight loss</u>, be sure to <u>reduce the number of calories</u> you consume. But, more importantly, make sure to eat <u>more quality nutrient-dense foods</u> and <u>less processed foods</u>.
3.	To avoid nutritional deficiencies that lead to chronic disease, nutrients should come from <u>whole foods first</u>, <u>then fortified foods</u>, and <u>last from supplements</u>. The exception is if you are prescribed supplements for medical reasons.

Chapter 2: At the Grocery Store

Shopping for the Right Food

We have already discussed how important diet is in maintaining overall health. However, all food is not equally healthy. For example, some food products are fortified or enhanced with nutrients, while others are loaded with natural or synthetic additives. In addition to some improvement in overall quality, these additives are often used to make the food more appealing for purchase by altering its appearance or taste. Some of these additives, however, can adversely impact health, especially if consumed excessively. In addition, the same food may contain potentially harmful chemical contaminates in trace amounts. Such contaminates are unintentionally added to the food during manufacturing and distribution. These are realities we have to deal with almost every day despite our best intentions to select the right types of food for our diet.

The concerns about added ingredients are legitimate. For instance, when we continually ingest processed foods, we may experience some form of inflammation (e.g. digestive problems) from certain ingredients that are mixed in them. Inflammation occurs when the body attempts to remove those foreign substances that are harmful or irritating in some way. The reaction gets worse the more we ingest and, even more severe, if we are overly sensitive to certain chemicals in the food.

Over long periods of time, constant exposure and gradual buildup of these ingredients can lead to chronic inflammation. And chronic inflammation has been linked to a variety of diseases. How do we know what food is safe? Product labels provide plenty of information, but understanding them is half the problem. This chapter will help clear up some of the confusion and provide insight into these labels, as well as address other concerns about safety in the grocery store.

When shopping, the potential **health problems** associated with selecting and consuming **the wrong foods** include the following.

• **Nutritional deficiency**, due to poor diet and inadequate nutrition, can result from choosing low-quality foods at the grocery store. This can potentially **increase the risk of chronic disease across the board**.

• Eating **too much of the wrong type of nutrient** can potentially **increase the risk** of chronic diseases and conditions such as **kidney disease**, **high blood pressure**, **heart disease**, and **obesity** [11].

• Chronic inflammation resulting from **overexposure to potentially harmful ingredients** can **increase the risk** of diseases such as **heart disease**, **diabetes**, **Alzheimer's disease**, **stroke**, **arthritis**, and certain types of **cancer** [32]. And, of course, chronic inflammation can also result from a food allergy or sensitivity to certain food additives.

*   *   *

It is therefore extremely important not only to make better food choices, but, also, to select the right (high quality) products when we walk down the aisle at the grocery store. In doing so, you will feel a sense of satisfaction knowing that you have made healthy decisions for yourself and for your family.

In this regard, to help prevent chronic disease and, otherwise, the incidence of illness, we can increase the nutritional quality of food we take home from the store through proper selection as follows.

• **Choose high quality whole foods**, as previously discussed, including nutrient-dense fruits and vegetables, whole grains, low-fat dairy products, and lean protein foods.

• **Identify the healthiest food products** by examining food nutrition labels and marketing labels that often appear on product packaging.

- **Limit the consumption of heavily-processed foods** that likely contain numerous food additives, including chemicals and other potentially harmful ingredients.

- **Limit the exposure to, and consumption of, known environmental contaminates** such as pesticides and other chemicals used to grow crops.

- **Eat a varied diet consisting of many different types of food** to reduce your risk of consuming high concentrations of some single contaminate that may be present.

$$* \qquad * \qquad *$$

We will address all of these key points and more. After reading this chapter, you will be able to avoid most of the potential health issues associated with shopping for food.

The Nutrition Facts Label

In the grocery store, the most important indicator of nutritional value comes from the "Nutrition Facts" label. This label is ubiquitous and appears on most packaged food to help shoppers determine how a particular food contributes to their diets. The current nutrition facts label, shown on the left side of figure 3, contains an abundance of useful information including serving size, calories, and the amount of certain nutrients such as fat, cholesterol, sodium, carbohydrates, and some vitamins and minerals. A list of ingredients is also included when appropriate. Examination of this label is a good starting point to evaluate what you are buying.

The Food and Drug Administration is proposing some minor changes to the nutrition facts label. You could see these new labels on food products in the near future (figure 3 on the right) [33].

Nutrition Facts

Serving Size 2/3 cup (55g)
Servings Per Container About 8

Amount Per Serving

Calories 230   Calories from Fat 72

	% Daily Value*
Total Fat 8g	**12%**
Saturated Fat 1g	**5%**
Trans Fat 0g	
Cholesterol 0mg	**0%**
Sodium 160mg	**7%**
Total Carbohydrate 37g	**12%**
Dietary Fiber 4g	**16%**
Sugars 1g	
Protein 3g	
Vitamin A	10%
Vitamin C	8%
Calcium	20%
Iron	45%

* Percent Daily Values are based on a 2,000 calorie diet. Your daily value may be higher or lower depending on your calorie needs.

	Calories:	2,000	2,500
Total Fat	Less than	65g	80g
Sat Fat	Less than	20g	25g
Cholesterol	Less than	300mg	300mg
Sodium	Less than	2,400mg	2,400mg
Total Carbohydrate		300g	375g
Dietary Fiber		25g	30g

Nutrition Facts

8 servings per container

Serving size   2/3 cup (55g)

Amount per 2/3 cup

Calories   230

% DV*

12%	**Total Fat** 8g
5%	Saturated Fat 1g
	Trans Fat 0g
0%	**Cholesterol** 0mg
7%	**Sodium** 160mg
12%	**Total Carbs** 37g
14%	Dietary Fiber 4g
	Sugars 1g
	Added Sugars 0g
	Protein 3g
10%	**Vitamin D** 2mcg
20%	**Calcium** 260mg
45%	**Iron** 8mg
5%	**Potassium** 235mg

* Footnote on Daily Values (DV) and calories reference to be inserted here.

Figure 3 – The current nutrition facts label is shown on the left. The proposed changes are shown on the right. Nutrients in the shaded area should be consumed in limited quantities (fat, cholesterol, and sodium are often over-consumed). Other nutrients, such as dietary fiber, protein, and vitamins, should be consumed in adequate amounts.

The proposed label accentuates the calorie count and number of servings to help with portion control. For both labels, however, nutrients in the shaded area should be consumed in limited quantities (fat, cholesterol, and sodium are often over-consumed). Other nutrients, such as dietary fiber, protein, and vitamins, are deemed essential to health and should be consumed in adequate amounts.

With only a few minor differences, both labels contain the following nutritional information [33, 34].

• **Serving size** – This is a standardized measurement (e.g. cups or ounces) to make it easier to compare the nutrient content of similar food products. Pay attention to serving size, as the rest of the label refers to nutrients for each specified serving of food.

• **Calories** – This is a measure of how many calories are in **each serving of food**. As previously stated, this is useful for portion control, and by extension, weight loss.

• **Total fat, cholesterol, and sodium** – Fat is a primary nutrient. However, to stay healthy, most of the total fat should come from unsaturated fats, such as those contained in olive oil and other vegetable oils. Be sure to limit intake of saturated fat and trans fat, as well as cholesterol (all in shaded area). An excess amount of these nutrients can increase the risk of certain chronic diseases and conditions, such as diabetes, heart disease, and high blood pressure [35].

• **Sodium** – Limit the intake of sodium (shaded area) to reduce risk of heart disease.

• **Carbohydrates** – Carbohydrates are a source of energy for the body. You should eat what is appropriate for your level of activity.

• **Dietary fiber** – Eat plenty of this plant derived nutrient for healthy bowel function.

• **Sugars** – Both labels show this nutrient, which can be consumed in its natural form (e.g. by eating fruit), or it can be consumed as an additive such as sucrose, high fructose corn syrup, or maltodextrin. The new label, shown in figure 3 on the right, deals with additives by including a category called "Added Sugars" (shaded area). Although there are no set guidelines for sugar intake, some diet plans still recommend limiting intake. And as you might already know, eating more sugar can dramatically increase calorie intake.

● **Protein** – You should consume plenty of protein. It is needed for energy and for building, repairing, and maintaining cells in the body.

● **Vitamins and minerals** – This section specifies some essential vitamins and minerals for health and includes, in the current label, vitamin A, vitamin C, calcium, and iron. You should get plenty of these in your diet. Under the proposed changes, vitamin D and potassium would have to be specified on the label. However, other nutrients, such as vitamin A and vitamin C would not, since these are no longer considered a serious problem in terms of nutritional deficiencies in the general population.

● **Ingredients list (not shown here)** – This section is included if the food product is made from more than one ingredient. If shown, it will appear immediately underneath the nutrition facts. Ingredients are always listed in descending order based on weight or concentration, with the higher amounts near the top. It is important to check this list for additives and other ingredients that may cause problems for those with food allergies or certain intolerances (more on this later).

Functional Foods

Some foods actually have additional nutritional value beyond what is normally found in its natural form. And then, there are some that are **perceived** to have additional health benefits. In both cases, their benefits may or may not be reflected in the nutrition facts label. However, they are often indicated on a marketing label or as a description in the name of the product. These foods are referred to as functional, a rather loosely-defined term.

Typically, there are three types of functional food when applied to added nutritional value. Although less than ideal, these foods can still help fill in nutritional gaps when whole foods are not available. Functional foods can be enriched, fortified, or enhanced [36].

● **Enriched foods** are those that are reconstituted to compensate for nutrient loss during processing. Food processing itself involves transforming the food into another form for distribution and consumption, and incorporates techniques such as mixing, de-aggregating, preserving, fermenting, pre-cooking, and packaging. To restore the nutritional value, the foods are enriched by artificially adding the nutrients back into the food.

● **Fortified foods**, such as breakfast cereals, contain artificially-added nutrients that are not normally found in the original or regular food. These nutrients are added to improve nutritional quality and improve overall health.

● **Enhanced foods** have nutrients added to them by modifying the food in some way, or by using indirect methods that are independent of processing. An example of an enhanced food is an omega-3 egg. The enhancement is done by feeding hens a large amount of flaxseed, which has high omega-3 fatty acid content.

$$* \qquad * \qquad *$$

As mentioned before, there are claims that some food contains health benefits that go beyond basic nutritional value. Although they may be considered functional, these claims are not assured. Often, they are supported only by the hope that some magical quality can reduce the risk of certain diseases, in addition to providing basic nutrition. Unfortunately, this is highly unlikely. Food is something not known to confer any additional benefits at all, beyond that of preventing nutritional deficiencies. Sure, a poor diet will lead to chronic disease, but that is why we choose healthy, nutrient-dense foods in general.

Marketers are aware of the trends surrounding these functional food claims. You'll notice that many of them use words and phrases like "this product may" or "possibly" when describing the benefit. That is the first questionable indicator. Alternatively, the described benefits may be extremely broad, such as "promotes heart health", "builds strong bones", or "promotes general well-being". This is done on purpose so the claims do not have to be substantiated. While all foods with nutritional value contribute in some way to these described benefits, there is nothing special about that particular food other than the presence and density of the nutrients contained within it.

You will also notice disclaimers near many of these health claims on the packaging [26]. This goes for many types of products, including supplements.

Example:

"This statement has not been evaluated by the Food and Drug Administration. This product is not intended to diagnose, treat, mitigate, cure, or prevent any disease."

These are telltale signs that the described benefits are likely exaggerated. Consider them as promotional acts only and take them with a grain of salt. Remember, the best way to get essential nutrients is through regular whole foods and not some special added ingredient. When that fails, you can still use enriched, fortified, and enhanced foods to help make up the difference.

Product Marketing Labels

Marketing labels, as opposed to nutrition labels, can mean different things. Even though they may have absolutely nothing to do with nutrition, we will pay more for certain foods because of them. Unfortunately, with so many of these labels, it can be difficult to choose the healthiest foods without overspending needlessly on false hope. Some of the more common ones are listed here with an explanation of what they actually mean.

If marked with an asterisk (*), the labels are significant in terms of health and nutrition.

General labels

● **Organic (*)** – Any product labeled organic has been produced without the use of synthetic pesticides, synthetic fertilizers, irradiation for preservation, or genetic engineering (referred to as genetically-modified foods or GMO foods). The organic label is regulated by the U.S Department of Agriculture (USDA), which essentially means that food producers and distributors undergo inspection and verification to make sure that the claim is accurate. If a product has a USDA Organic label on it, it comprises at least 95% organic content [37]. Foods that are organic can often be considered healthier than their non-organic counterparts, albeit more expensive to purchase.

● **Natural** – Unless the product has meat or eggs in them, the use of this label is not regulated and there are no standards regarding it. In other words, it could mean anything and should probably be ignored.

Meat and poultry labels

Note that most of these definitions have little to do with nutritional value or food safety [37].

● **Free-range** – This label means that animals were raised in some kind of shelter or enclosure, but with an opening to an outside area so they have access to fresh air.

● **Cage-free** – Animals were allowed to freely roam around some kind of shelter or enclosure that is big enough not to be considered a cage.

● **Grass-fed** – These animals were fed a grass-based diet during development, possibly supplemented with grain.

● **Pasture-raised** – Animals were raised with continuous and free access to an outdoor area for most of their lives.

● **Humanely-treated** – These animals were supposedly treated with care and compassion as they were raised. This label is not regulated by the

USDA and therefore carries little meaning, other than to make the consumer feel better about the process of producing the food.

• **Natural (*)** – Natural products are largely unprocessed and do not contain any artificial ingredients. Note that this term is **meaningful for meat, poultry, and eggs only** as opposed to its use in general, where it is not.

• **No added hormones** – This label also has little meaning as USDA regulations already prohibit the use of hormones or steroids in meat and poultry. The main purpose of this label is to differentiate a brand to make it more attractive on the shelf.

• **Brown eggs** or **White eggs** – There is no difference between white and brown eggs nutritionally. The change in color depends on the specific breed of hen producing them, and nothing else [38].

Fish product labels

• **Farm-raised fish** or **Wild fish** – Farm-raised fish are hatched, raised, and harvested under controlled conditions, whereas wild fish are harvested in the open water [39]. Both are considered healthy to eat.

Grain product labels

• **Gluten-free (*)** – The purpose of following a gluten-free diet is to treat a digestive condition called celiac disease, which affects up to three million Americans, or less than one percent of the population [40]. For others, gluten should not be a cause for concern. Therefore, any other health claims related to gluten-free products are debatable. In any case, grain products, such as wheat, rye, barley, and hybrids, which contain less than 20 parts-per-million of a protein called gluten, are labeled gluten-free as defined by the Food and Drug Administration.

● **Whole-grain (*)** – The term whole grain can refer to a number of different types of grains including whole wheat, brown rice, oats, barley, buckwheat, bulgur, millet, and corn [41]. Unfortunately, even with the label present, it can be difficult to determine how much of a product is whole grain and how much is simply refined flour and other ingredients. Check the ingredients label to verify that the grain is identified as a "whole" grain. If so, and if it is near the top of the ingredients list, there will be more of it in the product. A more convenient alternative is to look for the Whole Grain Council's Whole Grain Stamp (figure 4), which, if present, means the product contains at least 8 grams of whole grain per serving [42]. You can find additional information, including a list of products with the stamp, on the Whole Grain Council website.

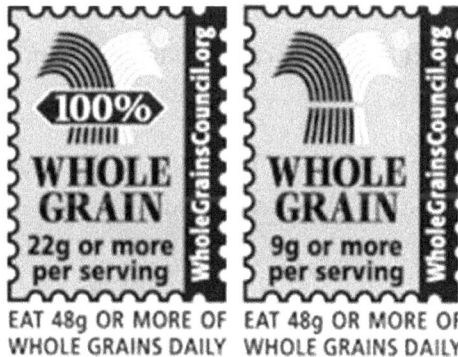

Figure 4 – The Whole Grain Council's Whole Grain Stamp. There are different variations. The 100% stamp (left) means all of the grain in the product is whole grain. The basic stamp (right) means some of the grains, but not all, are whole grains. There may be refined flour or other ingredients, such as extra bran, present in the product.

● **Multi-grain** – This label means the product has more than one grain. However, these grains do not have to be whole grains.

Nutrient specific labels

These labels describe the nutritional value of a product without having to give an exact amount of the nutrient in question. They are well-regulated and can be trusted to be accurate. As a form of marketing, they also make it easier to follow health guidelines or tailor diet plans, allowing shoppers to skip over parts of the nutrition facts label previously addressed [43, 44].

● **Low Calorie (*)** – One serving contains 40 calories or less. A meal or main dish contains 120 calories or less.

● **Low Fat (*)** – One serving contains three grams or less of total fat.

● **Low Saturated Fat (*)** – One serving contains one gram or less of saturated fat or can have no more than 15% of total calories coming from saturated fat.

● **Low Cholesterol (*)** – One serving contains 20 milligrams or less of cholesterol.

● **Low Sodium, Very Low Sodium (*)** – One low sodium serving contains 140 milligrams or less of sodium. Very low sodium contains 35 milligrams or less of sodium.

● **Reduced (*)** – This label can refer to calories, sugar, sodium, fat, saturated fat, and cholesterol. They appear as phrases such as "reduced sugar" or "reduced sodium". It typically means that one serving contains at least 25% less of a nutrient when compared to regular food.

● **Lean (*)** – One serving contains less than ten grams of fat, 4.5 grams of saturated fat, and 95 milligrams of cholesterol.

● **Extra Lean (*)** – One serving contains less than five grams of fat, two grams of saturated fat, and 95 milligrams of cholesterol.

● **Light (*)** – One serving contains at least a third fewer calories or 50% less fat. Note that this could also simply refer to texture and color depending on the context. For example, light could refer to light-colored bread.

● **Healthy (*)** – Generally, a healthy food is low in fat. One serving has 60 mg or less cholesterol, and 480 mg or less sodium. For many food types, they must also contain at least 10% of the daily value of one or more essential vitamins and minerals.

● **Free (*)** – Products that are labeled "fat free", "cholesterol free", or "sugar free" contain an insignificant amount of that nutrient. Note that the product can contain a very small amount of the nutrient and still be labeled in this way.

● **No Added Sugars (*)** – This label means that no sugar, or ingredient containing sugar, was added during processing.

*   *   *

The bottom line: whenever there is any doubt about a product marketing label, refer to the nutrition facts label (figure 3) for clarification. The nutrition facts label is well-regulated and very specific. It will tell you exactly what amounts are in the food (for the main nutrients) and include a list of ingredients. If a health claim cannot be explained by the nutrition label or isn't inherent to the type of food ingredient contained within, then the label is probably nothing more than a marketing term used to get your attention. Marketers know that the first product you look at on the shelf will probably be the one you take to the checkout counter.

Factors that Influence the Nutritional Quality of Food

When purchasing food products, especially fruits and vegetables, you want to make sure you are getting all the nutrients you expect from them. Unfortunately, there are a variety of factors that may adversely affect the quality of such foods. Consider how they impact nutrition, as follows [45, 46].

● **Processing and preservation methods** – There are a number of processing methods used to preserve foods. The objective is to maintain a similar level of quality to that of fresher counterparts. This is especially important for produce (e.g. fruits and vegetables) that is transported around the world. Different preservation methods such as canning, blanching or brief cooking, freezing, dehydration, pickling, and fermentation can all change the characteristics of food, including color, texture, and flavor. In most cases, these methods also decrease nutritional quality, especially when food is exposed to high levels of heat, light, and oxygen. So, minimally-processed whole foods, such as freshly-packed fruits and vegetables picked directly from the plant, vine, or tree, are likely to contain the most nutritional value compared to all other food in the grocery store.

• **Enrichment process** – As discussed earlier, it is expected that some nutrients will be lost during processing. That is why some foods are enriched through artificial methods to replenish those nutrients. As an example, milling (or grinding) removes much of the dietary fiber, vitamins, and minerals from cereal grains. Although enriching attempts to reintroduce some of those nutrients back into the food, it is simply not possible to replenish them all. This is a common problem with enriched white breads, for example.

• **Transport or storage for long periods of time** – Once a fruit or vegetable is removed from a tree, plant, or vine, it begins to degrade slowly. This degradation results in gradual loss of moisture, consistency, and nutrient composition depending on a number of variables, including how they are transported and stored. There is also a potential for spoilage. When examining fruits and vegetables at the grocery store, keep in mind the amount of time it took for the produce to get there, how long it may have been stored, and how long you intend to keep it before consumption. In terms of time, you may also want to think about where the crops were harvested. For instance, after inspection of the attached labels, you may find that some fruits and vegetables are imported from overseas.

• **Physical damage** – Mechanical harvesting techniques can cause stress to plant tissue and can damage the food in the process. The same damage can accelerate spoilage and nutrient degradation later on. Ideally, fruits and vegetables should be handpicked and handled gently.

• **Shelf life or freshness** – Shelf life, freshness-date, or use-by dates all give you an idea how long the particular food product has been stored or has been on display. Fruits and vegetables that have been sitting on a shelf for an extended period of time suffer the same drawbacks as those that have been in long-term storage. Nutrient loss is inevitable over time, especially if exposed to open air, light, and higher ambient temperatures. This also applies to meat and poultry, as well as other perishable items. Unless the food has been canned, frozen, or preserved in a way that allows for longer-term storage, chemicals will begin to break down the food fairly quickly and deterioration will occur. All of this will slowly degrade the nutritional quality of the food in question. Therefore, it is in your best interest to compare and select the freshest food option on the shelf each time you go shopping. That may mean looking in the back of the shelf for the newly-stocked products or verifying freshness with a grocery store clerk. Remember, the fresher the food, the more nutritious it will be by the time you eat it.

$$* \qquad * \qquad *$$

For these reasons, it is recommended to get as much food as possible, particularly fruits and vegetables, from local sources. **Local fresh markets** or **farmers markets** minimize the impact of processing, transportation, and storage on the nutritional quality of food. The produce sold at these markets is often harvested by hand and sold fresh shortly after harvest. Fruits and vegetables are going to be loaded with nutrients and will be quite healthy. It is no wonder that local markets are becoming more popular.

For a variety of other reasons, however, acquiring fresh, whole foods may not be an option. Or, access to a similar level of quality may be limited. Whether the circumstances are financial or geographic in nature, they should not prevent you from eating healthy. It is perfectly acceptable to rely on enriched, fortified, or enhanced foods to help meet nutritional needs. Although less than ideal, this type of food has been used around the world to maintain health and prevent chronic disease, particularly in areas where consistent access to whole foods is not available.

Food Additives and Health

A food additive is any substance that becomes part of the food for a specific purpose, typically before it is made available for purchase. This integration can occur at any time during processing, storing, and packaging of the food product. Not all additives are synthetic or man-made. For example, salt, sugar, and corn syrup are some of the most commonly used additives [47]. Although stigmatized in many cases, additives are quite useful and add to the quality of our lives. The following are some of the important uses of these substances [48].

• **To preserve food** – Preservatives are additives that help keep the food fresh over time to maintain quality, including nutritional quality, while it is distributed or stored. Preservatives prevent spoilage by limiting the proliferation of mold, bacteria, and yeast. They also prevent chemical reactions that lead to unwanted changes in color, taste, texture, and freshness; and, they prevent rancidity (foul taste or smell) as well. Examples of commonly used preservatives include salt, sugar, and chemicals such as benzoates, citric acid, and sodium nitrate [49].

• **To improve nutritional quality** – As previously addressed, additives can be used to fortify or enrich food products. Vitamins, minerals, and other nutrients are added to the food, in some cases, to make up for losses that occur during processing. In addition, with fortified foods, we can consume additional nutrients even if our regular diets are substandard. Examples of such nutrients include ascorbic acid (vitamin C), beta carotene (vitamin A), and calcium carbonate.

• **To improve taste and appearance** – Additives act as flavors, flavor enhancers, spices, coloring, and sweeteners. They can be natural (e.g. sweeteners such as honey, maple syrup, molasses, and agave nectar) or synthetic (e.g. aspartame, saccharin, and sucralose). The artificial ingredients tend to have deeper colors and stronger taste than their natural counterparts. Essentially, they improve the taste and aroma of food that we eat, making the process of eating more enjoyable. This has, without a doubt, improved all of our diets immensely.

● **To aid in processing of food** – Additives such as fat replacers, emulsifiers (for mixing), stabilizers, thickeners, binders, and texturizers (to improve texture and feel), leavening agents (for dough and batter), humectants (to retain moisture), strengtheners, conditioners, firming agents, and gases make food preparation easier. Because of these substances, food has the consistency and texture that is expected. Furthermore, with these additives, ingredients can be added (e.g. to fortify with nutrients) or removed (e.g. to reduce fat or sugar) so that we can get more of what we want in our diets.

*   *   *

Lately, it seems as if many additives have been unfairly categorized as unhealthy. This leads to an all-or-nothing attitude when it comes to certain ingredients. This is not necessary. Additives are regulated by the Food and Drug Administration, not to mention the food industry in general. They cannot be added if they reduce nutritional quality of food or if they are unsafe for consumption. All additives are investigated for safety and, therefore, many such ingredients have been deemed **Generally Recognized as Safe (GRAS).** Ingredients on this list have been extensively used in the past; or, if they are new, have been thoroughly researched and classified to have no known harmful effects. See the Food and Drug Administration website for the complete list of GRAS food additives [50].

Part of this confusion about the health of such additives is caused by reactions (in certain individuals) to the wrong food or certain ingredients added to the foods. Many of these reactions are rare, but word travels fast and fuels suspicion towards the ingredients.

There are two such reactions that can occur [51, 52].

- **Food allergy** – This is a reaction to food involving the immune system. It includes symptoms such as gas, headache, bloating, rash, hives, shortness of breath, and chest pain. Examples of common food allergy sources include peanuts, shell fish, eggs, wheat, and soy (table 6). In some instances, allergies can be life threatening, but, overall, food allergies are considered rare.

- **Food intolerance** – This is a gastro-intestinal discomfort that does not directly involve the immune system; however, it can have symptoms similar to allergies. Common symptoms of food intolerance include gas, diarrhea, headaches, joint pain, and constipation. Examples of food intolerance sources include lactose, sulfites, sodium nitrate, monosodium glutamate (MSG), and gluten (table 6). Most of these are food additives [53].

*   *   *

The list in table 6 is far from complete. After all, when it comes to food, there are a myriad of possible ingredients at play here. In any case, food intolerances are far more common than food allergies.

It is important to know what your sensitivities are and what you are allergic to. However, you should also realize that your condition is probably not related to some suspected toxic additive or some conspiracy theory involving regulatory agencies. If you are apprehensive over additives, the simplest solution is to drastically reduce intake of heavily-processed foods that have an abundance of such ingredients.

With this in mind, remember that the use of additives in moderation still carries a number of important benefits, and many additives influence health in positive ways. It is for this reason that we should learn to live with food additives and, when the situation calls for it, intelligently integrate them into our diets.

Common Causes of Food Allergies	Common Causes of Food Intolerances	
Egg	Gluten	Caffeine
Fish (salmon, tuna, halibut)	Lactose	BHA/BHT (preservative)
Milk	Sulfites	Aspartame
Peanut	Sodium Nitrate	Acesulfame-Potassium
Shellfish (shrimp, crab, lobster)	Saccharin	Artificial Flavorings
Soy	Olestra	Artificial Colors
Tree Nuts (walnuts, almonds, pecans)	Monosodium Glutamate (MSG)	
Wheat	Cyclamate	

Table 6 – List of common causes of food allergies and food intolerances. Food intolerances are far more common than food allergies.

Understand that just because an additive is natural, it does not necessarily make it safer than a synthetic or man-made ingredient. Both are chemically similar and both will have similar effects when it comes to consuming them in excess [54].

To reduce the impact of food additives in your diet, consider the following general guidelines.

● **Learn what causes your food allergies and intolerances** and stay away from those foods or ingredients (obviously).

● **Eat a well-balanced and varied diet**, as discussed earlier in this book. This will naturally and easily minimize the impact of additives and other substances in general.

● **Avoid eating disproportionate amounts of any particular food**, especially if you know they contain heavy amounts of certain additives. This is the case even if you believe they are non-toxic. For example, additives such as sugar, salt, corn syrup, dextrose, hydrogenated vegetable oil, mannitol, phosphates, plant sterol esters, polysorbate, sorbic acid, and artificial sweeteners all have the potential to cause unpleasant side effects and other health problems when consumed in excess [53].

● **Limit consumption of processed foods**, especially heavily-processed foods such as fried foods, sugary foods, and processed meats. This will also minimize the impact of additives and other hidden ingredients.

*   *   *

Note that if your diet is already healthy, you are probably already minimizing any negative impact of additives.

The key takeaway point is not to try to eliminate additives from our diet. Instead, **the key is moderation**. The objective is to reduce levels of added ingredients, whether natural or synthetic, to levels that remain beneficial from a nutritional standpoint, yet insignificant in terms of chronic disease.

Chemical Contamination in Food

There are hidden ingredients in our food that were not intentionally added and are referred to as contaminates. For example, in an industrialized society, the presence of trace chemicals and pollution in the environment is accepted as part of life. Contaminates, such as lead and arsenic, are also present all around us as part of nature, which may come as a shock. Other contaminates like synthetic pesticides and fertilizers are introduced into the environment to make our lives easier and more productive.

To some degree, then, all crops absorb chemicals and other contaminates whether or not they are grown organically. The problem with chemicals is that, after they are absorbed into our bodies or consumed at the dinner table, they are stored in fat, blood, and bodily fluids. The liver and kidneys, then, have to break them down to get rid of them [55].

Chemical substances can build up in muscle, bone, brain tissue, and other organs over time. These organs inevitably wear down, and, as we age, it gets more difficult to remove these chemicals from our bodies. For example, certain chemicals, like older pesticides, can stay in the system for many years [56]. They can even interact with other chemicals and each other, causing harmful reactions. Even trace amounts of a toxic chemical can result in chronic inflammation. And of course, at higher concentrations, the chemical burden will be much higher. Unfortunately, when some of these unwanted ingredients get into our food, they can, in some cases almost immediately, cause serious health complications for those with chemical sensitivities. And this can contribute to chronic disease.

There are thousands of chemical substances that can contaminate the food you are buying. Here are some general guidelines to avoid the worst of them.

● **Go organic for some fruits and vegetables** – Some fruits and vegetables are worse than others when it comes to pesticide contamination. Although organic food costs more, it may be worth spending extra to avoid such tainted produce. Table 7 lists the fruits and vegetables that typically contain the highest levels of pesticide residue [57].

● **Select fruits and vegetables that are free from visible damage** – If you select fruits and vegetables from the grocery store shelf that are free of cuts and other forms of damage, you reduce potential exposure to pesticides and other chemicals that may have leaked inside during production and distribution. Then, you can thoroughly clean the undamaged produce later to remove the remaining surface residue.

Apples	Kale
Celery	Nectarines
Cherry Tomatoes	Peaches
Collard Greens	Potatoes
Cucumbers	Spinach
Grapes	Strawberries
Hot peppers	Sweet bell peppers
Imported snap peas	

Table 7 – Fruits and vegetables that typically contain the highest pesticide residue. It may be beneficial to purchase organic varieties when dealing with these foods.

• **Limit fish consumption** – Pollutants in the water will be absorbed by fish in various quantities. For example, fish and shellfish (e.g. crab, lobster, clams, and oysters) can contain a toxic form of mercury, which can build up in the body over time when consumed. To minimize exposure to mercury and other chemicals, limit consumption of fish to **two or three servings per week** and white albacore tuna to about six ounces per week [58]. In addition, eat more salmon, shrimp, Pollock, light canned tuna, tilapia, catfish, and cod instead of shark, swordfish, tilefish, and king mackerel. This will also help limit mercury consumption. Lastly, when buying wild-caught fish, be sure to pay attention to fish consumption advisories.

• **Eat a variety of different types of food** – One of the best ways to minimize exposure to all chemical contaminates is to eat a variety of foods. This will limit the consumption of any one type of food with higher-than-normal concentrations. For example, all crops absorb arsenic to some degree, but rice typically absorbs more of it [59]. Of course, grains should be included in your overall diet. But, to mitigate the damage from arsenic even further, the solution is to eat a wide variety of grain products such as brown rice, barley, millet, oatmeal, whole grain bread, pasta, crackers, and wild rice. Note that seafood can also contain arsenic, so the same rule applies.

● **Eat a healthy diet** – If you are already eating lots of nutrient-dense foods, then you are also ingesting plenty of vitamins and minerals such as iron, calcium, and vitamin C. As it turns out, these nutrients will minimize absorption of certain chemicals, such as lead, in the digestive system [60].

● **Limit consumption of animal fats and organ meats** – Many chemicals are resistant to normal environmental degradation, and thus can be pervasive throughout the food chain. They first accumulate in animal foods through feed and water, and eventually make their way into humans. To reduce intake of these chemicals, we can simply eat less of the animal parts most likely to accumulate them [60]. Fat is the most common carrier, so be sure to purchase leaner meats that contain less fat in general. Also, reduce intake of products containing these fats, including margarine or butter, processed meats, and red meats. Try to rely on vegetable oils as a source of fat instead. Lastly, avoid or limit intake of animal organ meats such as kidneys and liver, as they tend to accumulate these toxins.

*   *   *

The bottom line for dealing with chemicals in food: eat a **well-balanced, varied diet consisting of as many different types of food as possible**. This will distribute the risk so that whatever you are ingesting does not increase your chemical burden or result in a toxic build-up over time.

Putting it All Together

In order to avoid chronic inflammation and nutritional deficiencies, we must not only follow a healthy diet, but we must also select the right foods when shopping. To accomplish this, we must study nutrition and marketing labels and understand what they mean. We must also understand what role additives play in our lives. Instead of trying to avoid them completely, we need to practice moderation by consuming them in limited amounts.

Additionally, we should recognize what causes our own food allergies and intolerances and understand that every individual is different and may react to food differently. We should also vary our diet by eating different types of food. That way, we spread out our risk of consuming an excess amount of chemical contaminates. This will also ensure that cumulative effects, beyond our bodies' capability to detoxify, do not increase to a level that is significant to long-term health.

Next, we will cover health as it pertains to food preparation and cooking. Even when making the right food choices, there are things we do in the kitchen that can negatively affect the nutritional quality of our food, as well as expose us to harmful substances.

Before proceeding, the following action steps can be taken right away to improve your health.

ACTION STEPS

1.	Understand and <u>refer to the nutrition facts label</u> on food products for information. Exercise caution with marketing labels, unless, of course, you fully understand what those marketing labels mean and can trust them as accurate.
2.	Purchase as much fresh food as possible, particularly <u>fruits and vegetables</u>, from local sources such as <u>fresh markets</u> or <u>farmers markets</u>. They will be loaded with nutrients and will be quite healthy.
3.	<u>Limit consumption of processed foods</u> to minimize the chance of unpleasant side effects from additives and other hidden ingredients.
4.	Eat a <u>well-balanced varied diet, consisting of as many different types of food as possible</u>. This will minimize concentrated exposure to chemical contaminates that may be present in food.

Chapter 3: Kitchen Basics

Food Preparation and Health

When we prepare food in the kitchen, we are essentially processing the food to make it ready for consumption. Food processing encompasses a number of different activities including cleaning, scrubbing, soaking, cutting, trimming, diluting, mixing, combining, and cooking. This is in addition to the processing that has already taken place from the moment the food is harvested to the time food is placed on store shelves.

Processing, and also food storage, can influence the nutritional value of the food we eat. Thus, these activities have the potential to influence our overall health. Previously, we discussed establishing a limit on the amount of heavily-processed food that we eat. By extension, if we process our own food excessively, we start to diminish its nutritional quality unintentionally.

The importance of diet in preventing chronic disease is clear. So, if the nutritional quality of food we eat is influenced by how we process food in the kitchen, then we should pay more attention to this activity. It is a commonly overlooked area.

But, simply focusing on the nutritional quality of food is not enough. Sometimes, toxic ingredients make their way into our food. For example, it is possible to inadvertently introduce chemicals into food during the food preparation process. Some of these chemicals are ubiquitous and nearly impossible to eliminate from our diet. In cases such as these, minimizing exposure may be the only solution.

Bacteria and other biological contaminates can also be a problem in an unsanitary kitchen. Since microorganisms are everywhere in our environment, it is important that we control their growth in order to limit excessive numbers of harmful variants in our food.

In the end, we need to maximize nutritional value and minimize exposure to unwanted ingredients.

The potential **health problems** associated with **excessive food processing** and **poor kitchen hygiene** include the following.

• **Nutritional deficiency**, due to poor diet and inadequate nutrition, is more likely when inadvertently lowering the quality of food during food preparation. This can potentially **increase the risk of chronic disease across the board**.

• Chronic inflammation resulting from **exposure to harmful ingredients** can potentially **increase the risk** of diseases such as **heart disease**, **diabetes**, **Alzheimer's disease**, **stroke**, **arthritis**, and certain types of **cancer** [32].

• Chronic inflammation is also possible with long-term **exposure to harmful bacteria** and other **biological contaminates** when operating in an unsanitary environment.

*   *   *

With this in mind, there are simple steps we can take in the kitchen to improve health. In reference to nutrient loss, the extent depends on a variety of factors, including the integrity of the particular nutrient involved and the time delay before consumption. Since the subject matter is so complex, this chapter will focus on basic concepts that can be more easily applied to help preserve the most important nutrients, while also ensuring that the food is safe to eat. It is not necessary to be perfect or stop enjoying food the way you like it. We will just bring some alternatives to your attention so you can get maximum nutritional value out of the food you purchase for your family.

Preventing Nutrient Loss during Processing

We know that food processing can alter or degrade the nutritional value of food. For nutrient-dense foods such as fruits and vegetables, this is obviously undesirable. Fortunately, there are a number of actions you can take right away in the kitchen to minimize this effect.

Consider, first, the following guidelines in reference to fresh fruits and vegetables [61, 62].

• **Eat as much of the whole food as possible** – We tend to throw away a lot more than we should. Unfortunately, some of the less palatable parts of fruits and vegetables may contain significant nutritional value. For example, apple peels, watermelon rinds, beet greens, turnip greens, potato skins, and pumpkin seeds are examples of healthy food parts that are commonly discarded.

• **Eat the outer layers when safe to do so** – A significant amount of nutrients are located in the outer layers of fruits and vegetables. For this reason, cleaning the surface is preferable to peeling or trimming when it comes to preserving nutritional value. If peeling is necessary, keep the extracted layer as thin as possible. To make it easier, you might use a fine vegetable peeler that is designed for this kind of work. You may also consider going organic for some foods, such as lettuce and cabbage, which are hard to clean. Organic produce will not have embedded pesticide residue, making consumption of the outer layers safer.

• **Leave fresh food intact until it is time to serve** – If possible, keep fresh food, especially raw fruits or vegetables, intact and untouched until it is time to serve. Peeling or dicing fruits and vegetables too early will expose the unprotected inner layers and accelerate degradation. Furthermore, dicing or cutting any food into smaller pieces increases the exposed surface area of that food to heat, light, and oxygen.

• **Don't clean vegetables by soaking them in water** – Water-soluble vitamins, such as vitamin C and B complex, and most minerals will dissolve in water. Therefore, try to avoid soaking vegetables in water before cooking. Instead, prepare vegetables with clean running water.

• **Consider blending rather than juicing** – When processing fruits and vegetables together into a liquid, consider blending rather than juicing, especially if you want to keep all of the nutrients intact. The process of juicing involves extracting liquid, leaving behind all the solids. While this juice will probably contain most of the vitamins and other nutrients contained in whole food, it does not contain all of them, and the juice will be missing a lot of fiber [63]. Blending, or mixing, whole fruits or vegetables together will create a liquid mixture of pulp, skin, and other plant matter, thereby providing a greater variety of nutrients.

*   *   *

Cooking, as another form of processing, can also affect the nutrient quality of the food being prepared. Although there is a belief that cooking will automatically reduce the nutrient quality of food when compared to eating it raw, this is not always the case. For example, some vitamins, such as vitamin C, are heat sensitive, while others, such as vitamin A, seem to be more abundant after cooking [64]. Such tradeoffs occur in all types of vegetables including carrots, spinach, mushrooms, asparagus, tomatoes, cabbage, and peppers. Naturally, the best way to take advantage of these health tradeoffs is to **eat a mixture of cooked and raw vegetables**.

There are a number of added benefits to cooking food, including preservation as well as improvement in digestion and taste. Here are some recommendations (e.g. for vegetables and meats) that help retain these benefits while reducing the amount of nutrient loss in the process [62, 65].

• **Use less water when cooking** – Microwave, steam, stir-fry, bake, or grill vegetables instead of boiling them in water. Boiling will result in loss of water-soluble vitamins such as vitamin C and B complex. Using the same logic, try to use as little water as possible no matter what cooking method is used. The exception is if you are ingesting the water as part of the meal. If you must cook the vegetables in water, consider saving the leftover water for use in soups, sauces, and juices. This extra water will contain the nutrients that were leeched during cooking.

• **Reduce cooking time and temperature** – Minimize the cooking time and temperature whenever possible. As stated earlier, too much heat destroys certain nutrients, especially the heat-sensitive vitamins (e.g. thiamine, vitamin C, and folic acid). So, when cooking vegetables on the stove, for example, cover the pot to hold in steam and heat. This will reduce cooking time. To reduce temperature, an effective alternative to cooking any food with high heat is to use a slow cooker. Even though it will take longer to cook, the temperature in a slow cooker is significantly lower and the lid is sealed, thereby preserving nutrients. This can also be quite convenient for food preparation since you can cook foods unattended without fear of overcooking.

• **Don't overcook** – Note that overcooking any food will reduce the nutritional benefit. It is important to cook meats long enough to kill any bacteria present; but it needs to be done using the lowest possible heat and shortest possible cooking time, while still being safe to eat. In the case of vegetables, they should be cooked until they are crisp or tender and then removed from heat as soon as possible.

• **Use the microwave oven more often** – Microwaving food is considered to be a superior technique for nutrient preservation when compared to roasting or grilling. Food will cook in the shortest possible time. Other methods may cook more unevenly and expose some parts of the food to excessive heat.

*   *   *

For all cooking methods, vegetables should be cooked just before serving to minimize nutrient loss from exposure to air. The bottom line for preventing nutrient loss when cooking is: <u>**minimize time**</u>, <u>**temperature**</u>, and amount of <u>**extra water**</u> used. In this regard, you should only use what is absolutely necessary to prepare the food for consumption. When choosing between any two methods of food preparation, choose the one that retains the most nutrients, and do it more often.

Preventing Nutrient Loss during Storage

A significant amount of nutrient loss occurs as a result of storage techniques. The longer a food is **exposed to air, light, and higher temperatures**, the more the **nutritional value decreases**, especially when it comes to sensitive nutrients such as vitamin A and C. It is therefore imperative that we pay attention to how food is stored, especially over the long term. This is especially true when we have already processed food for consumption and are saving leftovers for later.

The following are guidelines for maintaining the quality of stored food [66].

● **Eat fresh food as soon as possible** – When it comes to fruit, vegetables, and herbs, fresh (recently picked) produce is always better. Such produce loses nutritional quality the longer it is separated from the plant, vine, or tree. Therefore, try to eat fresh food as soon as possible for maximum nutritional absorption. Note that when you store food for later use, gradual degradation is inevitable in most cases. You can, however, slow down this process using preservation techniques (e.g. freezing).

● **Keep pantry food cool and refrigerated products cold** – Keep the pantry or food storage areas at a relative low temperature. Optimally, this is somewhere between 50 and 70 degrees Fahrenheit. Higher temperatures will accelerate degradation. Naturally, it is best to keep food storage cabinets and storage bins away from sources of heat such as ovens, hot pipes, or hot exhaust vents. Make sure any refrigerated foods are kept cold. Higher temperature equals faster degradation and changes in temperature will do the same.

● **Minimize exposure to air and moisture** – Use air-tight containers to prevent air and moisture from entering and degrading the product. Dry foods such as flour, crackers, cereals, cake mixes, pasta, seasonings, and canned goods should be stored in their original packaging if possible. This packaging is typically designed to help preserve food for transport. Alternatively, food can be transferred and stored in air-tight metal, glass, or plastic containers with tight lids. Make sure the rims and seals on all canned goods are protected. If they are damaged, the food will likely spoil.

● **Minimize exposure to light** – Use nontransparent packaging and containers (e.g. non-see-through plastic or dark glass jars) to minimize exposure to light. Any packaging that allows light will increase degradation depending on the type of food and other environmental factors. In general, store pantry food in dark areas. If there are windows in the room, use the added protection of bins, cabinets, or other larger containers to store food, especially when packaging itself allows air and light inside.

*　　*　　*

In a perfect world, we are able to acquire fresh food at precisely the time we are ready to consume it. Unfortunately, this is not always realistic. We need to be able to preserve food for longer periods of time, until we are ready to use it. To enhance the life of food, even beyond the recommended time limits, there are a number of different techniques available. Common examples include canning, dehydrating, and freezing.

As expected, there are trade-offs with such preservation methods, where some nutrients will be preserved while others will be lost [45]. For example, home canning uses heat or high pressure to kill microorganisms that degrade food. It naturally extends the shelf-life of food and preserves much of the nutritional value, but some heat-sensitive vitamins may be lost in the process. Dehydrating food will also reduce some of the vitamins due to exposure to dry and hot circulating air. But, it will increase other nutrients such as fiber due to the increased density of the final product.

<u>Freezing is an ideal method of preservation</u>. Freezing will preserve all the nutrients in a food product. This is a very safe method as long as a low temperature is consistently maintained and kept stable. Nutrient loss would only be expected before freezing, when the food is processed and handled, and then again, after freezing when the food is thawed and ultimately cooked.

The following are additional guidelines related to the freezing of food [66].

● **Minimize the time of exposure to high temperature** – If refrigerating or freezing leftovers, try to do so within two hours after cooking. Arrange space in the refrigerator around containers or packaging so that cold air can circulate and rapidly cool the food. You want to minimize the time food is exposed to higher temperatures.

● **Use the right packaging and containers** – When storing food in a freezer, use freezer-grade foil, wrap, or bags to protect the food. Ideally, containers should be moisture and vapor proof.

● **Make sure the freezing temperature remains stable** – Food quality will deteriorate at any temperature above freezing. Make sure the freezer temperature is sufficiently low to prevent this. If you are unsure about internal temperature, check to see if ice cubes are still frozen, or use an appliance thermometer. Note that temperature fluctuations can also cause degradation and further loss of nutrients. Therefore, it may be wise to avoid frost-free freezers for long-term storage applications. Additionally, make sure you have a sustained power source to avoid any partial or periodic defrosting during power outages.

*   *   *

Regardless of the food consumed, fresh foods tend to have the most nutritional value. The longer we wait to eat the food, the fewer nutrients it will contain. For food stored long term, we want to make sure the food is fresh enough to contain ample nutritional value and, more importantly, is safe to eat. Time stamp labels make this possible. However, the dates marked on packages can mean different things.

The following is a quick breakdown of these labels [67].

- **Pack date** or **Manufacture date** – This label refers to the date when the food product was packaged or processed for sale. These dates are useful for determining the overall age of the product.

- **Freshness date** or **Sell by date** or **Pull date** – This is used by the seller to determine how long to display the food product on the shelf for sale. The assumption is that this date allows buyers to consume the food at home within a reasonable period of time. The estimated time is typically determined by the manufacturer of the food product.

- **Use before** or **Best if used by** or **Best if used before** – This is the recommended shelf-life for overall quality. The food should be consumed before this date. However, if the food is preserved and shows no signs of spoilage, it may be consumed after this date.

- **Freeze by** – This indicates that the food product should be consumed, if not frozen for long-term storage, prior to the date shown on the label.

- **Expiration date** – This is the recommended last day a food product should be eaten. The exception is for eggs, which can generally be consumed up to several weeks after the date on the label [38]. For everything else however, the food should be discarded. This date also applies to emergency food, such as sealed dehydrated food.

*   *   *

It is a good idea to use your own labeling system for foods that do not have such dates marked on them. It should also be done for food products that are stored away for long periods of time, in case those dates fade or are wiped off somehow. When in doubt about the age of a food product, the safest thing to do is discard it.

Although first in, first out systems for consuming food from the pantry or freezer works for reducing waste, it may not be optimal when it comes to nutrition. With this in mind, be sure to **mix some fresh foods into your diet**, especially if you are consuming a significant amount from long-term storage.

Chemical Contamination in Food

There are traces of unwanted ingredients in our food despite our best efforts to shop for the safest food products. Unfortunately, there is no way to completely eliminate these ingredients from our diet as they are part of the environment in which we live. Although we have little control over the environment, we can still minimize unnecessary exposure once we bring the food home and prepare it. Consider the following guidelines to reduce the concentration of chemical contaminates in prepared food [60, 68, 69].

• **Remember to wash your hands** – Always wash your hands thoroughly before you prepare food. This cannot be emphasized enough. Hand washing will prevent possible contamination from ubiquitous chemicals, such as lead, and household chemicals, which may have been inadvertently handled throughout the day.

• **Remove parts of food that accumulate the most contaminates** – To reduce exposure to a number of chemicals in animal products, we can remove those parts that accumulate the most. This can be accomplished by trimming fat from meat and poultry, removing skin from poultry and fish, and discarding animal fats and oils from broths and pan drippings.

• **Avoid overcooked grilled food** – If cooking over a grill, burned portions of meat, fish, and poultry should be removed before consumption. Ideally, to prevent overcooking, consider precooking the food in an oven or microwave first, and then briefly grilling for flavor later.

• **Consider washing sealed containers before opening** – When stored in the vicinity of household chemicals, or near any toxic source, sealed food containers should be washed before you use them. This precautionary step will ensure that unwanted particles do not fall, or otherwise drift, into the food.

• **Wash all fruits and vegetables thoroughly** – To reduce exposure to pesticides and other chemical residue on the surface of fruits and vegetables, be sure to brush, scrub, and wash off all visible surface debris.

Such debris will probably contain the bulk of any residual contamination. Keep in mind that rough-skinned produce and leafy vegetables may have chemical residue in groves and crevices.

For some fruits and vegetables, you can peel or remove the outer layers. This will obviously remove chemicals on the surface. However, be sure to wash the outside of the entire food first to reduce risk of particles falling into the inside layers. The unfortunate tradeoff is that these outer layers are often the healthiest.

• **Consider discarding damaged fruits and vegetables** – If, after cleaning, you notice unexplainable damage or cuts in fruits and vegetables, you may not want to eat them raw, if at all. This damage provides easy entry points for pesticides and other chemicals into the food. In a sense, the natural barriers no longer exist. Keep in mind that even when there is no visible signs of damage, chemicals can still penetrate the outside layer of food. So, you won't be able to eliminate this risk entirely. But if you suspect heavy chemical or pesticide use, this would be further motivation for purchasing organic foods.

Note that more rigorous food preparation techniques such as cooking, freezing, dehydrating, and canning will also breakdown pesticides and other chemicals, thereby reducing the contamination level in the food. Again, the tradeoff is that these techniques may also reduce nutrient content.

*   *   *

In addition to chemicals in the environment, we can unintentionally contaminate our food over time through abuse, normal wear and tear, and corrosion of kitchen supplies, cookware, and storage materials. The end result is that trace chemicals (or higher concentrations) can end up in the food we consume.

Take plastic, for instance, which is common in the kitchen. All plastic containers leach trace amounts of chemicals into food (plastics contain chemicals). These can include phthalates and BPA (bisphenol A), depending on the type of plastic used. But, the amount is assumed to be small enough so as to not pose a known health risk. However, if we use the wrong type of plastic, heat any plastic beyond a safe temperature, or simply compromise the integrity of the material by damaging it in some way, then we risk introducing higher-than-normal concentrations of the material into the food we consume.

No matter what type of material we use in the kitchen, we should try to minimize exposure to the chemicals that are contained within it. To start, a simple rule of thumb is: **if the material is not clearly identified for storing, cooking, or handling food, then it should not be used in the kitchen**.

Now, consider the following general guidelines for safety when storing or cooking food.

When Storing Food

● **Store food in plastic containers designed for that purpose** – Plastic containers and materials that are sold in stores have a code printed on them for recycling purposes. This code tells you what types of chemicals are in the container (table 8) [70]. When it comes to reusing plastic containers to store food at home, number 1 and number 7 containers are ideal [71]. However, even though the type of plastic called PET (number 1) is generally safe to store food, the flimsy looking plastic bottles that are used to sell water and soft drinks are intended as single use only and should probably not be reused to store liquid [72]. Instead, use a plastic container that is **marketed as reusable**. HDPE (number 2) and LDPE (number 4) should probably not be reused as food containers or food liners. PVC (number 3) can be reused for food, however **make sure it was originally used to store food**. Plastic food-grade containers (number 6) are better used for temporary storage.

Plastic Codes	Type of Plastic	Food Containers
1	Polyethylene Terephthalate (PET)	Bottles for water, soft drinks, juice, sports drinks, beer, mouthwash, ketchup, and salad dressing; jars for peanut butter, jelly, jam, and pickles; oven films; microwave trays
2	High Density Polyethylene (HDPE)	Bottles for milk, water, and juice; grocery bags; cereal box liners
3	Polyvinyl Chloride (PVC)	Pre-formed packaging; shrink wrap; deli and meat wrap
4	Low Density Polyethylene (LDPE)	Bags for bread, frozen foods, and fresh produce; shrink wrap; stretch film; coatings for paper milk cartons; hot and cold beverage cups; container lids; squeezable bottles
5	Polypropylene (PP)	Containers for yogurt, margarine, takeout meals, and deli foods; bottle caps; bottles for ketchup and syrup
6	Polystyrene (PS)	Cups; plates; bowls; cutlery; hinged takeout containers; meat and poultry trays; rigid food containers; yogurt containers; loose fill peanut packaging; aspirin bottles
7	Other	Three and five gallon reusable water bottles; juice bottles; ketchup bottles; oven baking bags, barrier layers, and other packaging

Table 8 – Codes for plastics used to store and handle food. Note that if the material is not clearly identified for storing, cooking, or handling food, then it should not be used in the kitchen.

• **Instead of using plastic, consider substituting other materials** – For example, consider substituting glass, tempered glass (e.g. Pyrex), or ceramic containers whenever possible. Or use dishware (e.g. plates, cups, bowls, and casserole dishes) made of glass or stainless steel. These materials also hold up better to hot food.

When Cooking Food

• **Use reinforced or lined cookware** – When reinforced or lined cookware is manufactured, the metal is either made stronger, or it is lined with a harder one to prevent leaching into the food during cooking or other kitchen work. Examples include anodized aluminum and lined copper. Both of these metals are considered toxic if ingested in excessive amounts (reinforced or lined cookware prevents this). Note that any cookware made from stainless steel is fine on its own. There are no known issues with stainless steel as it is already very hard and resistant to damage, scratching, and corrosion. Cast iron is another exception and is also ideal on its own even though some rust may be present. This cookware may leach trace amounts of iron into the food, but this is acceptable since iron is considered to be an important nutrient.

• **Avoid using high heat with non-stick cookware** – Nonstick coatings are made from materials such as fluorocarbon, resin, and silicone. They can degrade and wear away over time, and may even chip off into food. Of course, newer materials are getting more and more resistant to this flaking. And, although the Food and Drug Administration claims that there is no health risk associated with ingestion of these materials, it is still advisable to minimize exposure when you can. This can be accomplished by avoiding excessively high heat (over 500 degrees Fahrenheit) and by not rapidly preheating an empty pan (a sudden temperature extreme). Basically, reduce the temperature to the lowest level you need to cook as discussed before. Also, when exposed to high temperature for long periods, non-stick coatings can give off fumes that are only slightly toxic. So, use the exhaust fan whenever you cook, for it will reduce the fumes released by this type of cookware especially when using certain cooking oils.

● **Avoid heating plastic in contact with food** – Consider removing the food from a plastic container, such as Tupperware, and heating it in a plate instead. If heating in the microwave, make sure the containers are microwave-safe at the very least. Note, even though a microwave oven does not heat the plastic of a microwave-safe container directly, it can still leach trace amounts of plastic into the food. The radiation will heat the food, which will then transfer heat back to the container during cooking and shortly afterwards. The reaction of elements in the food, combined with high temperature, may cause an interaction with the material in the container.

Whenever using a microwave, use paper towels, wax paper, or kitchen parchment paper instead of plastic wrap (table 8, number 3 and 4). Also, do not reheat takeout containers (table 8, number 5 and 6). These are intended for one time use and were only manufactured to transport food. Transfer the food to another container first. Finally, keep in mind that plastic (or nylon) kitchen utensils **melt when exposed to high heat**. Limit the amount of time they are exposed to any heat source, or use a safer alternative such as wooden or metal utensils.

● **Avoid abrasion when cooking or cleaning** – Be careful when using metal or hard plastic utensils on cookware, as they can cause scratches and abrasion. You do not want to wear down the metal lining in cookware. Instead, consider using wooden utensils when cooking.

Also, avoid using abrasive cleaning techniques, especially with materials such as steel wool. For plastics, consider washing containers by hand rather than by machine, as it will reduce the risk of damage. If a plastic container or metal pan is damaged (e.g. cracked) or worn, you may not want to use it to store or prepare food. Weakened material may expose the food to increased chemical residue.

*　　*　　*

Remember, when using cookware, the bottom line is to **avoid excessively high heat and abrasion**. Both can compromise the integrity of the materials used to cook and expose the food to chemicals.

Biological Contamination in Food

All food contains a certain number of microorganisms (e.g. bacteria). However, we still need to minimize risk of ingesting too much of the wrong type. Doing so can be detrimental to health in the short-term by leading to food poisoning. In the long term, however, an unsanitary environment can continue to expose us to higher concentrations of harmful microorganisms over and over again. Regardless of how the microorganisms got into the food, when their presence is unwanted and harmful, the food is considered contaminated.

The following are common sense strategies that should be employed when preparing food to reduce risk of biological contamination [73, 74].

• **Remember to wash your hands before handling food** – Always wash your hands thoroughly, with soap and water, before you prepare food. Do not be concerned about the temperature of the water from the kitchen sink, for it will never be hot enough to kill bacteria. It is more important that you use soap, and that you rub your hands together vigorously to dislodge any particles on the surface of your hands [75].

• **Clean and sanitize all food preparation surfaces** – Make sure food preparation and cooking surfaces are clean and sanitized. Keep in mind that something can look clean, but not be sanitized. By sanitizing a surface, almost all microorganisms are removed or killed. So, after you thoroughly clean a surface by removing dirt and food scraps (using soap and water), sanitize it with a kitchen sanitizing product such as chlorine bleach, hydrogen peroxide, or white distilled vinegar. Be sure to leave it on the surface for the recommended amount of time. The same should be done with utensils if you don't plan on using a dishwasher. If you are using disinfecting wipes, do not use the same wipe on multiple surfaces, as this may spread contamination.

● **Cook all meat, poultry, and eggs thoroughly** – All meat, poultry, and eggs should be thoroughly cooked. When broiling or baking meats and poultry, you may want to use a thermometer to make sure that the food is cooked throughout at a sufficient temperature. The minimum safe temperature for cooking most food is around 165 degrees Fahrenheit. Eating raw meat, poultry, and eggs should be considered risky. If not cooked, they may contain dangerous amounts of Salmonella, Listeria, or other harmful microorganisms.

● **Be careful not to cross-contaminate** – To avoid cross contamination, keep raw meats separate from fruits and vegetables. Avoid the temptation to rinse raw meat and poultry before cooking them, as the water may contaminate another surface in the process. Be sure to clean and sanitize cooking utensils and cutting boards after processing poultry and meat. Do not prepare other food using the same tools and surfaces unless they have been sanitized. Also, do not put cooked food in a dirty container that previously held raw meat or poultry. In general, make sure you keep such foods separate from all other food and each other unless you are in the process of cooking them. Lastly, be sure to wash your hands thoroughly with soap and water afterwards.

● **Wash all fruits and vegetables thoroughly** – This is especially important if you are eating them raw. Brush, scrub, and wash the produce to remove visible surface debris, as discussed earlier in the chapter. Note that bacteria can be mixed with debris and lodged in areas that are difficult to access. Consider peeling or removing the outer layers of rough-skinned produce or leafy vegetables if surface contamination, biological or otherwise, is suspected. Naturally, cooking will kill residual microorganisms.

● **Refrigerate leftovers as soon as possible** – Lower temperatures will slow down the growth of microorganisms. Alternatively, use proper food preservation techniques such as freezing or canning to prevent further growth.

*   *   *

It can be difficult to determine if food is unsafe due to the presence of harmful microorganisms. After all, we can't see them. However, in many cases, spoiling food displays visible and recognizable signs that a dangerous amount of bacteria or toxin may be present. For example, unusual odor, color, texture, bubbling, foaming, or the presence of scum could all be signs that spoilage has occurred. If you encounter such signs, it may be safer to discard the food in question, rather than to risk illness [76].

Note that for meat and poultry, color alone may not indicate spoilage. For these foods, color changes, such as a greenish color in meat, can be common. Even if you can find discolored meats for sale, this does not mean the food is bad. However, if, in addition to color change, you notice an unusual odor or a slimy texture on the surface, then it is likely unsafe to eat [77]. The food is also unsafe even if it is cooked afterward. Simply discard it. A bout of food poisoning may pass in the short-term, but exposure to harmful microorganisms from unsafe food may complicate health in other ways later.

Putting it All Together

We covered how food preparation in the kitchen affects overall health. This is an area that we often overlook. And it does have significance when it comes to our diets. In so many cases, we have to strike a balance between preserving the nutritional value of food and reducing exposure to harmful ingredients. Perfection is not possible nor is it necessary. Compromising between nutrition and exposure depends on our health, our chemical sensitivities, the environment in which we live, the availability of food, and the resources we have in the kitchen.

The safest bet in almost all circumstances is to try to introduce as much variation into your diet as possible. Use a mixture of fresh and preserved food products. Use various food preparation techniques and cooking methods. This will not only ensure that you get a variety of nutrients in your diet, but it will also minimize potential exposure from high concentrations of harmful foreign ingredients that are consumed too often in one type of food.

By slightly changing the way we do things in the kitchen, we can be sure that the food choices we make are contributing to our overall health, the way we expect them to. And it doesn't have to take too much effort.

The following action steps can be taken right away to improve your health.

ACTION STEPS

1.	When it comes to eating fruits and vegetables, consume <u>as much of the whole food as possible</u>. Additionally, <u>consume a mixture of raw and cooked vegetables</u> to take advantage of the health tradeoffs that are present with each preparation method.
2.	Don't overcook. When cooking, <u>reduce time and temperature to only what is needed</u> to serve the food and make it safe to eat.
3.	When storing any food, <u>minimize exposure to air, light and high temperature</u>. Eat fresh food as soon as possible, as it contains the most nutrients.
4.	For both cooking and storage, only use materials that are <u>clearly identified for handling or storing food</u>.
5.	<u>Clean the kitchen regularly,</u> and don't forget to <u>use a kitchen sanitizing product</u> such as chlorine bleach, to remove and kill all microorganisms on food preparation surfaces. This is especially important when dealing with raw meat and poultry.

Chapter 4: Exercise and Physical Activity

The Importance of Exercise and Physical Activity

One of the major risk factors of chronic disease and disability is lack of physical activity. So, naturally, one of the easiest ways to counteract that risk is to move more. A regular exercise program is one of the greatest tools at your disposal for improving overall health and longevity. Unfortunately, many people don't use it. When an exercise program is recommended, some individuals probably visualize spending hours at the gym most days of the week. However, this is totally unnecessary unless you plan on becoming a professional athlete. For most people, such a goal is unrealistic. Amazing health benefits can come from small durations of exercise every week, and it doesn't even need to occur at a gym.

Exercise is a great preventive tool to combat a wide range of chronic diseases and related conditions, for it strengthens our body and mind in so many ways. This benefit alone makes following a consistent exercise program an imperative, regardless of your level of fitness or when you start. There are many secondary benefits to overall quality of life as well.

Exercise and regular physical activity have the following **health benefits** [78, 79]:

- **Prevents** unhealthy weight gain and **obesity**

- **Reduces risk** of **heart disease**

- **Reduces risk** of **type 2 diabetes**

- **Reduces risk** of many types of **cancer**

- **Strengthens** the **musculoskeletal system** (e.g. bone, muscle, tendons, and ligaments) so we can stay mobile for longer

- Improves our peak bone health which **prevents osteoporosis**

- **Improves mental health** and mood

- **Prevents** falls and other **accidents** caused by daily activity

- **Improves overall health** and **increases longevity**

*   *   *

There are potential **short-term benefits** as well. For example, you may notice a **boost of energy** after a few weeks of exercise. You will probably be able to think more clearly during the day and **manage stress** more effectively. Among other noticeable benefits, exercise may **keep you from getting sick** as often. Do you have trouble sleeping? Exercise may also help you get **better quality sleep** at night.

For those who are well-informed on this subject, many of these health benefits are obvious. However, many people still do not engage in regular exercise, let alone enough physical activity to maintain the recommended baseline for health. By definition, physical activity is any sustained movement of the body that burns more calories than simply sitting on the couch. This doesn't seem too difficult, right? It could be in the form of walking, doing housework, playing sports, or going to the gym. The widespread lack of such activity is at least partially responsible for the obesity epidemic in the United States that is so often discussed in the media. And it is getting worse.

As we become more occupied in our everyday lives, not having a plan to address this shortcoming can make incorporating some form of physical activity into our schedules quite difficult. This is unfortunate in that it does not take a rigorous exercise program to accomplish what is needed.

Instead of overcomplicating what should be an easy fix, we should strive to do at least the minimum amount of physical activity required to maintain health. We do not have to be gym fanatics, although that would be admirable if one has the time. Remember, though, in the case of exercise, more is not always better. If we can schedule small blocks of time to do some form of physical activity, and stick to it like we would a business appointment, we would have a better chance at maintaining a decent level of consistency.

As stated previously, exercise and physical activity are critical to preventing chronic disease. It also makes us even **more resilient to unrelated illnesses**. This will be especially true later in life. In fact, exercise is becoming so important that some scientists are considering highlighting such data on food labels in lieu of the number of calories per serving [80]. Doing so would encourage people to look at food differently. Instead of focusing on counting calories all the time, food choices would be influenced by each individual's exercise schedule or by a certain expected level of physical activity on a daily basis.

Aerobic Exercise

There are several ways to get exercise. One way is through aerobic activity, which is any activity that improves your endurance. It involves longer-term sustained movements using larger muscle groups or the entire body. Examples of such activities include walking or swimming. Aerobic exercise is good for strengthening the cardiovascular system (the heart and blood vessels), which no doubt helps to prevent, and otherwise mitigate, heart disease (or cardiovascular disease). The U.S. Department of Health and Human Services has outlined what we need to do when it comes to aerobic activity [81]. This is a good starting point no matter what your fitness goals are. If one is living a largely inactive lifestyle, or is not exercising at all, these guidelines need to be followed at a bare minimum.

Aerobic activity can be performed at the gym, playing sports, or even doing outdoor or home improvement work. Some vocations may be very physical in nature (e.g. masonry, carpentry, construction, or moving services) and would also qualify as exercise. So, if your job is already labor intensive, you are probably getting most of the exercise you need for the week.

Not all exercise is equal, however. Depending on your level of fitness, you may be able to do higher-intensity exercises, which will require less time. If you are out of shape or have a condition that prohibits you from performing certain types of activities, you may only be able to do low or moderate-intensity exercises. Determining the intensity of exercise is relative depending on factors such as age, fitness level, and how much effort you are really exerting personally. Naturally, if you can perform higher-intensity exercise, you'll need less of it per week to stay healthy. When the intensity of exercise is lowered, however, more of it is required.

We will start with explaining what you need to do for moderately-intense exercise.

On a side note, the health benefit of exercise does in fact depend on duration. You would not experience the same health benefits if you only did one or two minutes of exercise at a time. So, that simply means walking around the house for a few minutes will not qualify. The rule of thumb is that an activity must take **at least 10 minutes at a time** for it to be valid.

*   *   *

Moderate Intensity – In general, you are doing what is called moderately-intense aerobic activity if you can continue to hold a conversation while you are working up a sweat. For an idea as to what is typically considered moderate activity, see figure 5 [82]. Examples that fall under this category are listed in order by number of calories burned in 30 minutes. So, the more intense exercises are closer to the top of the list, while the less intense exercises are closer to the bottom.

Moderate Intensity Exercises

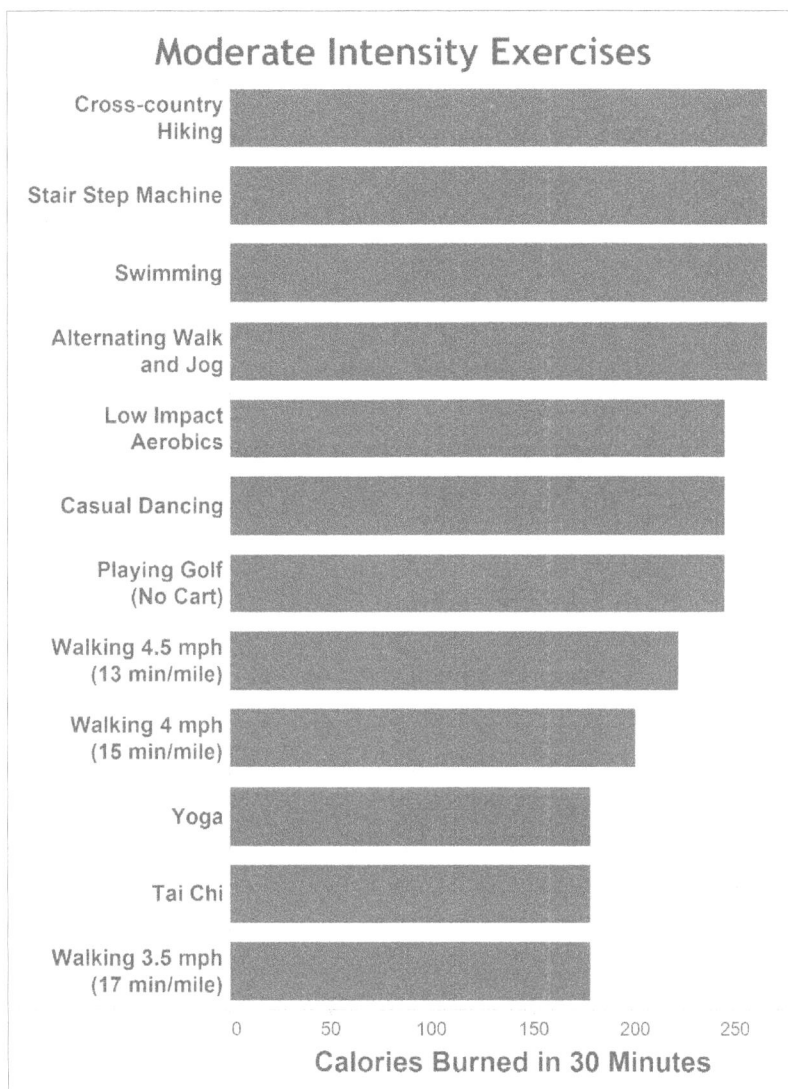

Figure 5 – Examples of moderate-intensity aerobic activities. They are listed in order from higher intensity to lower intensity based on the number of calories burned in 30 minutes. These numbers refer to calories burned by an average person weighing approximately 185 pounds. The exact number of calories burned will vary for each individual.

According to standardized physical activity guidelines for health, the amount of recommended moderate-intensity exercise is as follows.

• **Good** – You should exercise a minimum of **150 minutes or 2.5 hours per week** according to your schedule. For example, you could do 50 minutes of walking per day, 3 times per week, or spread it out even further by doing 30 minutes of walking, 5 times per week.

• **Better** – For increased health benefits, including weight loss, you could do **300 minutes or 5 hours per week** according to your schedule. For example, you could do 60 minutes of walking per day, 5 times per week or you could try splitting it up during the day by doing 30 minutes of walking in the morning and 30 minutes of walking at night.

*   *   *

Anything over 300 minutes per week would be considered highly beneficial for health if it is within your capabilities. However, this is not required. Keep in mind, also, that more exercise is not necessarily better for your health. It depends, in large part, on your fitness level. If you are not in good shape or are consuming too few calories for your level of activity, you can experience sickness more often, as well as suffer from symptoms of overtraining (e.g. chronic fatigue). This will not make you healthier. In fact, it may do the opposite by increasing joint inflammation and possibly lead to injury.

Regardless of fitness level, individuals should strive for a recommended 150 minutes of any activity a week, engaging in those that are safe and fun. Being a minimalist in this fashion will probably increase your chances of sticking with a regular program, especially if you are short on time.

For the most benefit, exercise should be spread out over most days of the week (e.g. 4 or more days). An example schedule is shown in table 9 with various types of moderate-intensity aerobic activity, which you can modify according to availability of facilities.

Sun	Mon	Tue	Wed	Thu	Fri	Sat
10 min Walking		10 min Walking	10 min Walking		10 min Walking	
10 min Walking	Resistance Bands	20 min Stair Step Machine	10 min Walking	Resistance Bands	20 min Swimming	30 min Hiking
10 min Walking			10 min Walking			

Table 9 – An example schedule for 150 minutes of exercise per week. This schedule combines moderate-intensity aerobic exercise with strength training (e.g. resistance bands).

Notice that on some days, exercise is split up throughout the day in shorter increments. Do whatever your schedule allows; just be sure to get the minimum 150 minutes. And be sure that each session is at least 10 minutes in duration.

*   *   *

High Intensity – When you are engaged in high-intensity aerobic activity, you are breathing hard and not able to say more than a few words at a time before pausing to take another breath. With this level of exercise, you would not have to commit as much time to achieving long-term health benefits. In fact, you can reduce time spent on overall aerobic activity to half of what was done on a moderately-intense exercise program.

To illustrate, figure 6 lists examples that fall under this category by number of calories burned in 30 minutes [82]. As in the previous figure, more intense exercises are closer to the top, while less intense exercises are closer to the bottom of the list.

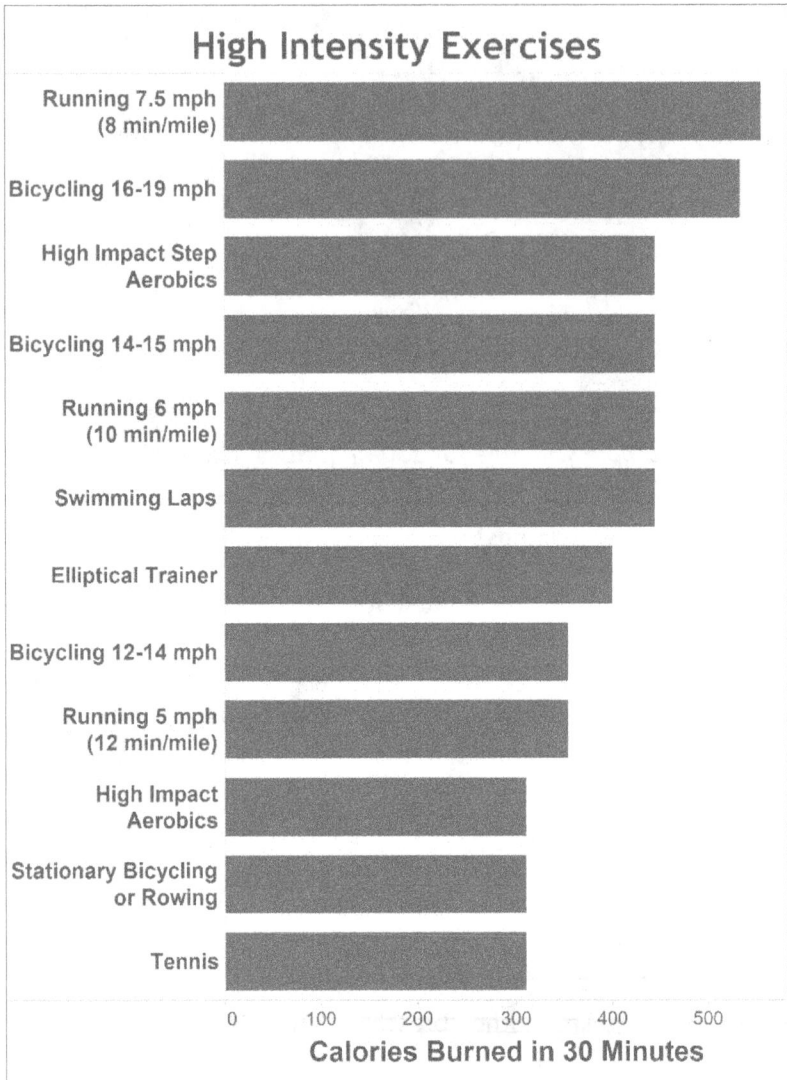

High Intensity Exercises

Running 7.5 mph (8 min/mile)
Bicycling 16-19 mph
High Impact Step Aerobics
Bicycling 14-15 mph
Running 6 mph (10 min/mile)
Swimming Laps
Elliptical Trainer
Bicycling 12-14 mph
Running 5 mph (12 min/mile)
High Impact Aerobics
Stationary Bicycling or Rowing
Tennis

0   100   200   300   400   500

Calories Burned in 30 Minutes

Figure 6 – Examples of high-intensity aerobic activities. They are listed in order from higher intensity to lower intensity based on the number of calories burned in 30 minutes. These numbers refer to calories burned by an average person weighing 185 pounds. The exact number of calories burned will vary for each individual.

According to standardized physical activity guidelines for health, the amount of recommended high-intensity exercise is as follows.

● **Good** – For high-intensity exercise, you should exercise a minimum of **75 minutes or 1.25 hours per week**. For example, you could do 25 minutes per day of running, 3 times per week, or spread it out even further by doing 15 minutes of running per day, 5 times per week.

● **Better** – For increased health benefit, including weight loss, you could aim for **150 minutes or 2.5 hours per week** of exercise. For example, you could do 30 minutes of bicycling per day, 5 times per week or split up activities during different parts of the day. These are just examples.

*   *   *

Anything over 150 minutes per week would be considered highly beneficial for health if you feel comfortable doing it. Again, be careful not to overdo it. If you notice you seem to be going backwards in terms of performance or fitness progression, you could be overtraining.

Try any split that you want, as your schedule allows, as long as each session is 10 minutes or longer in duration. Another example schedule is shown in table 10, this time with various types of high-intensity aerobic activity, which may be modified according to availability of facilities. Create your own schedule and split up your activities so they are spread out over most days of the week. Just be sure you get the minimum amount of exercise. Follow some type of exercise schedule and stick to it week after week. You can change up activities, but you must be consistent. Our goal is long-term health and so our bodies will need time to adapt to a fitness program.

Sun	Mon	Tue	Wed	Thu	Fri	Sat
30 min Tennis	Weight Lifting	20 min Running 10 min Stationary Rowing	30 min High-Impact Aerobics	Weight Lifting	20 min Running 10 min Stationary Rowing	30 min Bicycling

Table 10 – An example schedule for 150 minutes of exercise per week. This schedule combines high-intensity aerobic exercise with strength training (e.g. weight lifting).

Strength Training

Most people should integrate strength training exercises into the overall exercise program at least twice a week to collectively reinforce bone, muscle, tendons, and ligaments.

Strength training is any exercise that involves lifting weight or pushing and pulling against some form of resistance. Note that it does not have to involve iron weights. For example, some sports such as wrestling, rowing, gymnastics, and even swimming have a strength training component inherent in the activity. For those who don't play sports or engage in such activities, there are also a number of alternatives to lifting weights at the gym. Resistance bands, suspension straps, and elastic cables are some examples. This type of apparatus is available on the market and can be set up at home or almost anywhere.

Ideally, a strength training program should involve working various muscle groups using moderate or high-intensity effort as follows [81].

● Perform strength training at least **two times per week**. Table 9 (e.g. resistance bands) and table 10 (e.g. weight lifting) are examples of how one might incorporate strength training into a complete workout program. You should schedule a day or two between strength training workouts to prevent overtraining and allow for muscle recovery.

● Include major muscle groups such as the legs, hips, back, chest, abdomen, shoulders, and arms. At minimum, try to train each muscle group at some point during the week. If you are short on time, choose exercises that work more than one muscle group at a time.

● Each exercise should involve at least 1 set of a certain number of repetitions, typically 2 or 3 sets are considered more effective. Aim for around 8-10 repetitions per set. An example of a repetition is 1 pushup. Depending on fitness goals, the number of repetitions can vary.

● Use the amount of weight that is safe for you. In other words, keep the amount of weight or resistance to a level that matches your usual level of activity. If you can exceed that level, increase the amount of resistance **gradually** to avoid risk of injury. Give your body time to adapt.

*   *   *

Note that, unlike aerobic exercise, there is no recommended amount of time for strength training activities. The amount of time will vary depending on the exercises performed and the number of sets and repetitions.

Other Physical Activities

Sometimes performing high and even moderate-intensity exercise can be difficult. In this case, it is advisable to get as much exercise as possible depending on your unique circumstances and whatever stage of life you are in. As such, older adults are encouraged to do whatever they can, whereas children are encouraged to do more than the recommended amount to improve growth and development.

Even if you can't do any such strenuous activity, you need to do something. Keep in mind that some of the perceived strenuous activities, such as swimming, are lighter on the joints and may be well within your capabilities. For other conditions (e.g. chronic pain), a healthcare practitioner, such as an exercise physiologist, may be able to help find activities for your unique situation.

Don't just give up completely. Any amount is better than nothing at all. If scheduling time to exercise is a daunting task or finding a suitable location to get it done is near impossible, there are still other options. Some activities that you engage in may already be considered exercise. If this is the case, do more of it! For example, many regular household chores and outdoor activities burn as many calories as gym exercises. Many of these activities tend to get overlooked for their health benefits. Increasing such activities is a unique opportunity to do something useful while exercising at the same time.

In figure 7, some common household chores, outdoor activities, and home improvement tasks are listed according to calories burned in 30 minutes [82]. Notice that some of them could be considered moderate or even high intensity! For comparison, if you are sitting down, doing desk work, or watching television, you would be burning anywhere from 30 to 80 calories every half hour.

Even if you are sitting at a desk or working on the computer for hours on end, there are products on the market that allow you to increase physical activity while you work. Some examples are desk exercise bikes (less expensive) and standing desk treadmills (more expensive). If you are creative, there is almost always a way to get the required amount of exercise in for the week. It is important to note, that some light activities such as cleaning the house or dusting furniture may not amount to any significant level of exercise when compared to a regular exercise program.

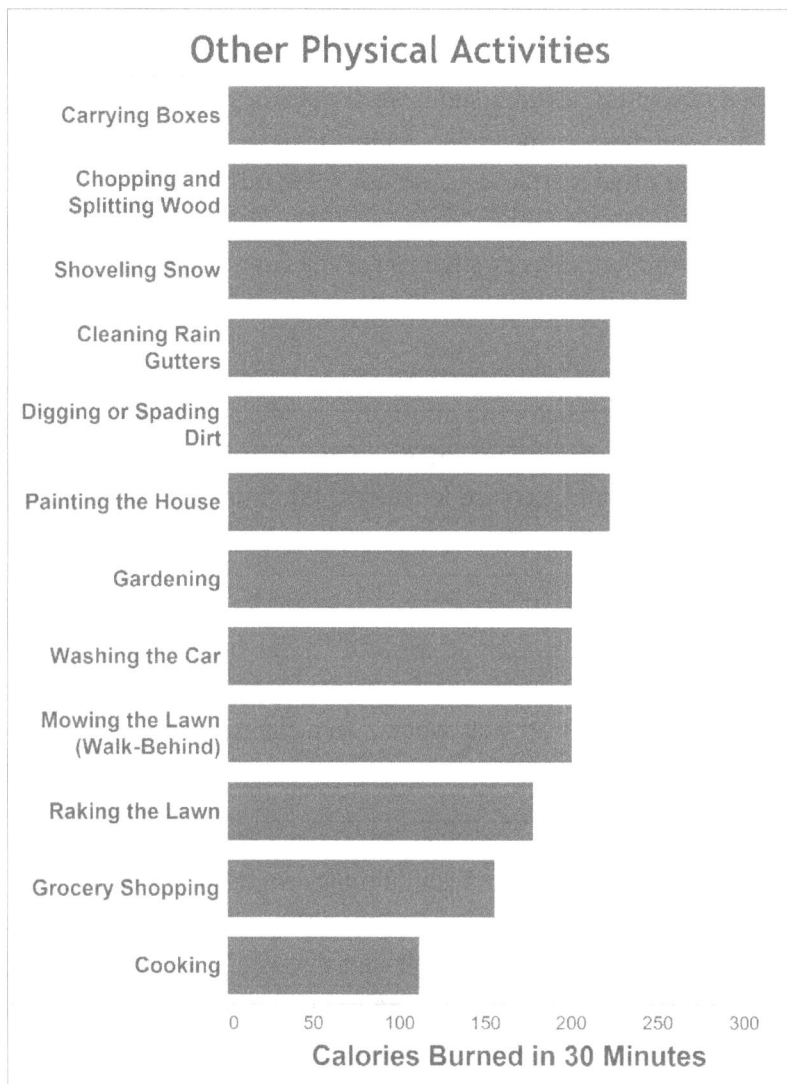

Figure 7 – Examples of other physical activities that fall outside of what is normally called exercise. Some of these household chores and outside work activities qualify as moderate-intensity or even high-intensity exercise. All of these activities are better than simply sitting down or doing nothing at all. The numbers here refer to calories burned by an average person weighing 185 pounds. The exact number of calories burned will vary for each individual.

Lifestyle-Related Physical Activities

To achieve maximum health benefit, we should try to get as much physical activity into our lives as possible. Unfortunately, thanks to advances in technology and other distractions, we are going outside less and on top of that we are sitting down more. These bad habits are making it harder to get even the minimum amount of physical activity we need each day, let alone the exercise we need for the week.

Luckily, there are some subtle ways we can squeeze even more activity into our lives without too much extra effort. For example, by simply standing up and moving around throughout the day, even as we work in an office, we improve our health and increase longevity [83]. Sure, this may not qualify as the recommended level of exercise as stated earlier, but it will still help in the long run.

Other methods are so easy that we don't even have to put it into our schedule or set aside a special time for it. Some may actually work as mini-exercise sessions, as a short walk would. To achieve a more active lifestyle, consider the following guidelines.

● **Do more walking** – The next time you drive anywhere, try parking your vehicle a little farther away than you normally would to get in a short walk. The same goes when taking a bus. For example, exit a block or two farther from your destination. Or, when walking somewhere in a large building or around a campus, explore a bit and take the longer way around. Try not to be in a hurry all the time.

● **Climb more stairs** – Take the stairs rather than the elevator, even if you can only manage a few floors at a time.

● **Take more active breaks** – While at work, take short breaks to walk around, stand up, or stretch. This is especially important for those that work at a computer desk all day. For example, one study suggests that older adults should take as many as nine such breaks per hour [84].

- **Spend more active time with family and friends** – Instead of just sitting around, catch up on events with family and friends while taking a walk together outside. Alternatively, if the weather is bad, move this activity indoors to someplace like a shopping mall.

- **Spend more active time with your pets** – Pets can help improve your health. You know how any dog feels about a walk outside. So, from this incentive, find time to walk the dog regularly, even if it is for a short while.

- **Try out a new active hobby** – Consider adopting relaxing new hobbies that involve more physical activity. As one example, people of all ages can take ballroom dance classes to learn a new skill and meet new people.

- **Play more physical video games** – If you spend a lot of time playing video games already, try to play more physical games on platforms that use motion and gestures rather than a handheld controller. This is also called exergaming.

*   *   *

As you can see, these activities do not take a major commitment of time, money, or effort, and they can be enjoyable. Remember that it is in your best interest to stay active by any means necessary. And maintaining mobility throughout life is critical. So, get creative and come up with your own lifestyle-related physical activities. You have probably heard this before: if the activity is simple, convenient, and fun, you are more likely to stick with it over the long term.

Putting it all Together

The key takeaway point is that no matter what condition you are in, try to incorporate as much exercise and physical activity into your life as you can. This not only helps prevent chronic disease, but will also strengthen the body to help cope with health challenges encountered later in life. Think of a strong body as a buffer against potential chronic diseases and disabilities.

A strong body will also keep you mobile much longer and that is a major key to living longer and maintaining a positive state of mind.

Obviously, if you have not exercised in a long time, it may be prudent to get a physical checkup beforehand. Not only will this ensure you start a new exercise program safely, but you will probably get some additional advice from your healthcare provider. Depending on your situation, this may help you remain physically active in a variety of ways over the long-term.

Remember also, no matter what exercise program you start, increase intensity slowly. This is common sense. If you do not give your body time to adapt, you risk injury. And, of course, you cannot maintain proper health if you are injured.

Finally, before you begin to procrastinate, take action now to improve your health!

ACTION STEPS

1.	Schedule <u>a minimum of 150 minutes</u> of <u>aerobic exercise</u> each week. Make sure it is spread out <u>on multiple days</u> during the week.
2.	Schedule some kind of <u>strength training</u> on <u>2 or more days</u> during the week. You can integrate it into any existing exercise program.
3.	Come up with <u>a few lifestyle-related physical activities</u> and incorporate them into your daily routine. Be creative. Keep it simple. This is in addition to regular exercise.

Chapter 5: Sleep and Stress Management

The Dangers of Lack of Sleep and Excessive Stress

The importance of sleep is often overlooked when it comes to long-term health. It is at least as important as other preventive measures such as diet and exercise. So often, however, the never-ending demands at home and at the office cause many of us to shun sleep as something that gets in the way of productivity. This is unfortunate as sleep is absolutely essential to warding off chronic disease.

When we lose out on sleep, we do not simply catch up by squeezing in more of it on the weekends or during time off. Each night we get an insufficient amount of sleep, we place an undue burden on our entire body. Obviously, this can lead to noticeable complications in the short-term and affect overall quality of life. However, the problems do not stop there. Lack of sleep is implicated in more serious medical conditions and even influences other risk factors, such as unhealthy weight gain and obesity [85]. Quite simply, if we do not get this condition under control, the adverse effects of sleep deficiency will accumulate over time. And such problems tend to catch up with us in the form of chronic disease later on.

Another byproduct of the lack of sleep is enhanced susceptibility to stress on our bodies when we are awake. Stress can originate from other factors as well, such as persistent worry or exhaustion from excessive labor, as examples.

Stress and lack of sleep are interrelated. To illustrate, if you don't get enough sleep, you are likely experiencing increased stress. If you are stressed, you probably aren't getting enough sleep. This cycle can obviously feed on itself and make conditions worse.

This is why both subjects are covered together in this chapter. Furthermore, we need to address both conditions in order to effectively decrease our risk of chronic disease.

The potential **health problems** associated with **lack of sleep** include [8, 86]:

● **High blood pressure**

● **Increased risk** of chronic diseases and other conditions, including **diabetes** and **heart disease**

● **Increased risk** of **accidental injury**

● Weight gain leading to **obesity**

● Development of **mental and emotional problems**, including depression and anxiety disorders

● **Increased stress**

*　　*　　*

The potential **health problems** associated with **excessive stress** include [87, 88]:

● **Impaired immune function**, which increases risk of illness

● **Increased risk** of chronic diseases and other conditions, including **diabetes**, **heart disease**, and **cancer**

● Development of **mental and emotional problems**

● Musculoskeletal disorders and **increased risk** of **accidental injury**

● **Inadequate sleep**

*　　*　　*

Stress, as a temporary condition, is not necessarily a bad thing. It is essentially a reaction of the body to change. We use this reaction to solve problems and cope with temporary hardships. On the other hand, if stress is chronic and excessive, our bodies will never have a chance to recover properly. This is what contributes to long-term health problems and chronic diseases.

You should notice that many of the health problems associated with lack of sleep and stress are, as listed above, nearly identical. This highlights the close relationship between them. Both conditions can be difficult to deal with depending on the circumstances. However, sleep disturbances are often easily identifiable and thus, are easier to remedy. Stressors, on the other hand, can be very subtle and difficult to pinpoint. For this reason, we'll start by addressing sleep.

Without sleep, you cannot hope to manage stress.

How Much Sleep Do You Need?

To start, exactly how much sleep do you really need? This has been the subject of debate. Not only is the number of hours important to each individual, but the quality of that sleep is extremely important. If you are not getting quality sleep, you could be getting less overall sleep than you think, even if you spend more time in bed.

As a guideline, when it comes to hours of quality sleep, less than six hours has been found to be detrimental to health. Conversely, getting too much sleep, in excess of nine hours, can be unhealthy as well [89].

The general recommendation is that somewhere between seven and eight hours of sleep is adequate for adults. Some studies indicate the magic number for longevity and health is **between 6.5 and 7.5 hours per night** [90]. This appears to be a good target range for our busy lifestyles.

Note that this does not apply to children. Children typically need more sleep than adults. It is critical during early development.

Factors that Can Affect Quality of Sleep

It may seem easy to schedule a certain number of hours of sleep and feel as though the issue of sleep has been dealt with. However, there are other factors at play when it comes to sleep quality, and they vary for each individual. Some factors can be controlled and some cannot, but all must be taken into consideration when addressing sleep.

The following factors affect the quality of sleep [91, 92]. Note that any one factor or a combination of factors has the potential to reduce the amount of quality sleep to a dangerous level.

• **Age** – As we get older, we are more at-risk when it comes to health problems that affect sleep. Some of these problems manifest as sleep disorders such as insomnia, which is quite common in the elderly. Others simply reduce our ability to get uninterrupted sleep. Although we can expect our sleep patterns to change as we age, we need to anticipate these changes and adapt accordingly.

• **Gender** – We obviously can't do much about this on our own. For example, in women, menopause can make sleep difficult due to changes in hormone production.

• **Sleep schedule** – An erratic sleep schedule can affect our circadian rhythm, which is when our body expects to go to sleep and when it expects to wake up. When we change our sleep schedule abruptly, we interfere with our body clock and, as a result, may have trouble sleeping. In most cases, though, we have control over this issue.

• **Lifestyle** – An inactive lifestyle (e.g. little to no exercise) can make sleep, especially quality sleep, more difficult. This holds true for other ill-advised lifestyle choices such as smoking and excessive drinking.

• **Medications** – Medications almost always have side effects. Obviously, you need to be aware of what medications you are taking right before bedtime. But, even medications taken throughout the day can affect sleep if they have long-lasting effects.

- **Medical conditions** – There are a number of medical conditions, including many of the chronic diseases covered in this book, which can affect sleep in one way or another. Unfortunately, most of these associated sleep problems cannot be corrected without some form of medical treatment to control the underlying cause. If not corrected soon, any reduction in sleep quality can actually make these conditions worse.

- **Environment** – Any unnatural condition that disrupts sleep needs to be regulated. This includes sound, light, and temperature. Even if you do not wake up, a disruption from your surrounding environment can make six hours of sleep seem more like three, while keeping you in a state of constant restlessness. Fortunately, we can largely control these conditions.

- **Surgery** – The invasiveness of surgery, along with associated anesthesia and other medications, can affect sleep adversely. And it can take a while to recover from this level of trauma and return to a normal sleep routine.

- **Sleep disorders** – Whether brought about by an underlying medical condition, or not, there are a number of disorders that affect sleep. Some common ones include sleep apnea (breathing disruption), restless leg syndrome, insomnia, and narcolepsy (sleep-wake cycle disruption). Like other medical conditions, these may have to be corrected by some form of medical treatment.

- **Behavior** – Some abnormal behaviors could be considered sleep disorders and most are correctable. An example is late-night eating which can be detrimental to sleep if done immediately prior to bedtime or throughout the night.

- **Mental state** – An unhealthy mental state such as depression can make sleeping difficult. Many such conditions are influenced by stress. Others may require treatment.

- **Stress** – This is related to our mental state and can interfere with sleep patterns. We will cover stress later in this chapter.

* * *

For the factors that you can't control, you either have to compensate by increasing the overall hours of sleep or you may need to seek a medical solution. Whichever method you choose, be sure to address the problem as early as possible.

Now, let's discuss common sense actions to overcome some of these limiting factors.

Guidelines for Better Sleep

There are a number of things you can do to get more sleep, as well as improve the quality of sleep. If you cannot correct a sleep problem in short-order, it is best to consult your healthcare provider or a specialist as quickly as possible to identify and fix the problem. The longer you wait, the more you risk compounding a lack of sleep with other health problems that may surface as a result.

The following best practices and guidelines may help you get more quality sleep [93, 94]. As long as you are not suffering from a medical condition or disorder that prevents you handling sleep problems on your own, try these out and see if you feel more energized and rejuvenated the next day.

Sleep schedule

● **Follow a consistent sleep schedule** – Try to go to sleep and wake up at approximately the same time each day. If dealing with factors outside your control such as changing shift schedules or extensive travel, make adjustments to stay as close as possible to your original sleep schedule. Otherwise, try to ease into a new one over time. To help adhere to an existing schedule, consider following a regular evening ritual that relaxes you. For example, taking a warm bath, listening to soothing music, doing some easy reading, or meditating each night will establish a pattern that will help your body prepare for sleep.

Environment

● **Control Sound** – Be sure to sleep in a quiet room. Make sure there is no noise or sound disruption during sleep. In other words, try not to sleep with the radio or television on all night long. If you have a partner who is a loud snorer or who grinds his or her teeth at night, consider ear plugs, noise cancelling electronics, or soothing sound makers to help drown out the disrupting noises. Also, put your cell phone away, on silent mode, to avoid interrupting calls if you expect them.

● **Control Light** – Be sure to sleep in a dark room. Consider using shades, blinds, or curtains if the room is too bright from outside light sources. This is especially important if you have to sleep during the day. Use a low-wattage night light to maintain room orientation if you anticipate having to get up in the middle of the night. Too much light all at once, perhaps from a table lamp, may keep you from going back to bed. Additionally, be sure to turn off electronics, bright screens, or anything that produces significant ambient light during the night. Such light will fool the body into thinking it is time to wake up.

● **Control Temperature** – Sleep in a room that isn't too hot or too cold, and ensure that the local temperature will stay stable throughout the night. If the temperature cannot be controlled, obviously you will need to make adjustments using more or less clothing. If your feet are cold, put on loose-fitting socks. If your head is cold, use a knit cap. Both the feet and head will radiate heat throughout the night. Therefore, if both are covered to retain heat, the rest of your body will stay warm as well.

Lifestyle

• **Exercise regularly** – Stay physically active throughout the day and get the recommended amount of exercise you need each week for general health. Lack of physical activity can exacerbate sleep problems. In addition, musculoskeletal problems caused by lack of exercise can result in debilitating and sleep-depriving pain. This measure requires more time to work, which is why it is listed as a lifestyle remedy.

Medication

• **Double-check medication** – It may be possible to change the way you take medication by modifying the dosage, time of day, or even the type of medication that you suspect is interfering with a regular sleep pattern. To start, you should check the labels on over-the-counter medications to confirm you are using them properly. If you are, you can try substituting other medications or adjusting the dosage schedule when feasible. If the medication is prescribed, you need to consult your healthcare provider before making any adjustments. Keep in mind that some over-the-counter medications such as pain relievers, diet pills, and cold remedies contain stimulants which can interfere with sleep.

Medical conditions

• **Acquire better sleeping apparatus** – If you suffer from pain that interferes with sleep, consider acquiring a mattress that provides better support and body alignment. Firm mattresses are generally the best option for proper back support, although those preferences vary from person to person. As an alternative, use inner knee cushions, leg and head support pillows, and inflatable bed wedges to help you deal with the pain more effectively.

• **Try alternative medicine techniques** – Consider incorporating alternative medicine techniques to help alleviate symptoms associated with a medical condition. For example, aromatherapy (e.g. using essential oils such as lavender), meditation, massage therapy, or hydrotherapy (e.g. taking a hot bath), could be effectively used in this way [95]. The evidence may be lacking as to the effectiveness of such treatments for general health, however, if it helps you relax, alleviates symptoms of a medical condition, or promotes better sleep, those methods are worth exploring.

• **Preserve your teeth** – If you have a tendency to grind your teeth at night, it may also be disrupting your sleep. If your dentist has not already created a mouth guard for you, consider acquiring one to wear throughout the night. If anything, it will also help preserve your teeth.

Behavior

• **Stop using electronic devices** – If you are accustomed to reading with electronic devices before bedtime, consider substituting these e-readers, tablets, or phones with traditional books, when the situation allows for it. The blue light from these devices may fool the body into thinking it is daytime. At the very least, turn the brightness setting down as low as possible. On a related note, you may want to avoid certain stimulating forms of entertainment before bedtime (e.g. watching action programs on television).

• **Avoid taking naps** – If you do nap, do not take one too late in the day, since it may interfere with normal sleep. Keep naps short, no more than half an hour if possible. If you find that you have problems falling asleep later on, try cutting out the naps completely.

• **Relax** – Refrain from working, or engaging in overly stimulating activity, within 30 minutes before bedtime. Use that time to wind down. Do something relaxing, such as reading or listening to music. This will also help reduce stress, which is detrimental to sleep. As an alternative, try other techniques such as meditation and stretching exercises (e.g. yoga) to help you relax. Any activity that is enjoyable, slows you down, or otherwise provides minimal stimulation should do the trick.

• **Exercise earlier in the day** – Avoid exercising within two hours of bedtime if you find such activities interfere with sleep. For some, however, this may actually promote sleep. In general, though, it is best to exercise earlier in the day.

• **Don't force it** – If you cannot fall asleep within twenty minutes or so, consider getting up briefly and then trying again a short time later. Whatever activity you do in the meantime, make sure it is not overly stimulating as mentioned before.

• **Watch what you eat late in the day** – If you must snack late at night or in the middle of the night, avoid heavy, spicy, or sugary foods, which, for some individuals, may adversely affect sleep.

• **Watch what you drink late in the day** – Cut back on fluids later in the day. Excessive fluids may increase the need to urinate in the middle of the night. Avoid caffeine, nicotine, beer, wine, and liquor at least four to six hours before bedtime. Caffeine in particular can remain in your system for up to seven hours [96]. Keep in mind that many drinks contain caffeine, including coffee, tea, sodas, cocoa, and hot chocolate. Note: foods that contain chocolate can also have caffeine. As for alcoholic beverages, you may be thinking, from previous experiences, that they can help you sleep. This is a misconception. Although it can encourage a light sleep initially, alcohol actually prevents you from achieving deeper stages of sleep, and that is what is necessary for health [95].

*　　*　　*

If it is safe to do so, you may try over-the-counter sleep aids. Realize that there are side effects to such drugs, including behaviors similar to sleepwalking, or even allergic reactions. Be sure to follow product instructions and warnings on the label [97]. Keep in mind that this type of medication is intended only for temporary use and is by no means a permanent solution to an underlying sleep disorder or medical condition.

When attempting to self-diagnose sleeping difficulties, it may be helpful to keep some sort of written or electronic journal. In this journal, record the time you go to bed and time you wake up. Include details such as what you had to eat and what activities you were engaged in before you went to bed. Keep track of various environmental factors as well. Trying to pinpoint factors that contribute to your sleep problems, as opposed to an underlying medical condition, is difficult without some way to track what is going on. Even if you end up seeking medical help, a journal will enable your healthcare provider to more effectively diagnose and treat your sleep-related condition.

These recommendations may not work for everyone and they are not, by any means, universal. The only way to know for sure that something works for you is through trial and error. But, do try, for you may be surprised at what you can do for yourself.

Next, we will cover how to manage stress to improve health. Not surprisingly, doing so will also help us sleep better.

Recognizing the Signs of Stress

As stated earlier, stress can have long-term health ramifications if left unchecked. A byproduct of persistent stress is exposure to other chronic disease risk factors. For example, stress can lead one to indulge in excessive alcohol consumption, smoking and tobacco use, as well as recreational drug use and other distractions. Additional risk factors only compound the problems that stress already causes, so it is imperative to get stress under control as soon as possible.

It is important to remember that we cannot completely eliminate stress. Not only is it part of life, but it is beneficial in a sense that it helps us adapt to change and handle new challenges. What is important is that we control it so that it does not become excessive or chronic in nature.

To be able to cope with stress, whether it is short-term or long-term, you must first learn to recognize the symptoms. Stress can manifest in subtle ways, slowly building up over time. And, dealing with day-to-day problems, including interpersonal conflicts, can exacerbate the stress we are already experiencing. Even though the signs may not be obvious at first, you must be observant and aware to spot them in the early stages. Table 11 lists some of the symptoms that are commonly associated with stress [98].

Signs of Stress		
Difficulty sleeping	Disbelief and shock	Indecisiveness
Being angered easily	Tension	Feeling numb
Feeling depressed	Feeling anxious about the future	Losing interest
No desire to eat	Recurring thoughts about event	Irritability
Depression	Feeling loss of control over life	Headaches
Stomach problems	Back pain	Trouble staying focused
Experiencing unusual fatigue		

Table 11 – Common signs of stress. In order to cope with stress early, we must learn to recognize the signs.

By recognizing these symptoms early, you can be proactive in interrupting the pattern or behavior that causes them. That is, by addressing these problems early, you avoid dangerous and more challenging conditions later.

Also, it is not good practice to wait until others tell you that you appear to be under a high level of stress. Doing so may make the stressful conditions worse than they need to be. You are responsible for yourself. Stay aware, stay educated, and stay in active control over your own mental state.

Remedies for Mitigating Stress

There are a number of things we can do on our own to deal with stress. Naturally, as large as this topic is, we cannot discuss every aspect of it. Also, since coping with stress is a bit of an inexact science, many of the potential remedies are subjective in nature and may not be effective for everyone. This makes universal guidelines difficult to compile. However, information that is presented here is more than adequate as a starting point for development of your own coping mechanisms.

The following are some common sense practices and guidelines for preventing and coping with stress [98, 99, 100].

Preventing stress

• **Maintain good health through diet and regular exercise** – A healthy body can enable you to resist the effects of stress more easily than if you are in an unhealthy state. Be sure to maintain a healthy diet and do exercise regularly. As discussed earlier, healthy habits established now can pay dividends later, not only in allowing you to resist chronic disease, but also in coping with stress more easily in the future.

• **Get adequate sleep** – As covered earlier in the chapter, getting adequate sleep will reduce stress and lessen the effect of future stressful situations on the body in general. You cannot adapt to stress effectively if you are sleep-deprived or worn out. On the other hand, using excessive sleep as a tool to avoid or escape the realities of stress is also not recommended.

● **Normalize your work schedule** – Working too many hours over time can lead to increased stress, decreased productivity, and other chronic conditions. It is acceptable to push hard for a deadline every once in a while. However, if you commit to working too many hours week-after-week or month-after-month, you are at risk of becoming more vulnerable to stress during hard times. So, instead of working more than eight hours a day, try to be more productive during your existing work hours. Studies have shown that every hour you work over eight hours will decrease productivity anyway.

● **Plan ahead and rehearse** – Plan for stressful lifestyle changes ahead of time. If you expect to encounter stress (e.g. a semester exam, switching jobs, or moving to a new area), then you are already aware of what is coming and you can take steps to prepare. You may even consider imagining bad outcomes in your mind's eye and how you would maneuver around and away from them. Don't try to ignore them, and don't schedule anything else that can compound the level of stress you are likely to experience during that time.

● **Be a minimalist and simplify your life** – Consider adopting a minimalist lifestyle in areas most likely to introduce new stressors. In a sense, you need to rid yourself of distractions that are unnecessary, counterproductive, and likely to lead to a stressful state in the future. As a typical example, always keep your work area clean and well organized. From this author's experience, it is a powerful way to buffer against being completely overwhelmed by unfinished demands when new work comes your way or new challenges reveal themselves.

● **Spend less time worrying about news of current events** – If the news of current events bothers you, reduce your intake to a level that is more comfortable. It seems like the media focuses only on bad news these days, therefore learn to break regularly from the news. Simply turn off the television and radio and ignore current events that you cannot control anyway. Also related, when you read the newspaper early in the morning, the bad news can set a negative tone for the whole day and magnify upcoming stressors.

• **Improve communication with others** – In many situations, this is the best remedy to prevent stressful situations. This way, you can work out all kinds of differences early when they are small, thus avoiding unnecessary conflict. For example, on the job front, you can reduce stressors by communicating with associates to resolve issues related to excessive workloads and looming project deadlines.

• **Be realistic about what you can accomplish** – Realize your limitation as a human being and try not to be over-ambitious. Be realistic about what you can accomplish and learn to say no more often, before you become overwhelmed. Be confident that you can easily avoid this form of self-inflicted stress. Furthermore, when you do have to accomplish a task that is perceived to be too large and potentially beyond your capabilities, whittle it down by going after the smaller and simpler tasks first. So to speak, the way to move a mountain is to start with the smaller hills and then with a shovel if that is all you have. At this point patience and persistence will almost always provide you with success eventually.

• **Stay positive and adjust your attitude** – Learn to stay positive in the face of adversity and be confident in your own abilities. Use this strength of character to be more aware of and more knowledgeable about the stressful issues in your life. In doing so, you will be more prepared to control and mitigate potential stressors in the future.

• **Follow a daily routine** – Try to maintain a normal daily routine. This kind of discipline will give you a solid mental baseline and you will be able to better cope with changes brought on by new stressors. Too much change at once can create a more stressful environment and lead to a feeling of hopelessness.

Coping with Stress

• **Don't self-sabotage** – During stressful times, avoid the temptation of indulging in self-sabotaging behaviors such as drinking or using drugs. Recognize that these vices can potentially make stress worse later on and will further increase the risk of chronic disease in the process. Also, don't further agitate your nerves by overdoing coffee and sugar. Just follow a healthy diet to provide your body with adequate nutrition and energy.

• **Prioritize and reduce your load** – Handle the most important tasks first. Decide what needs to get done now and what can wait until later. Procrastinate on those things that don't matter as much. If you are already experiencing stress, don't add to it with additional stress that could have been prevented or delayed. And don't multitask. In other words, don't try to tackle any new challenges until the one you are dealing with is under control. Focus on one thing at a time.

• **Take breaks and don't forget to exercise** – Consider occasionally taking a break from what you are doing to gather your thoughts for control, clarity, and stress reduction. One easy option is to go outside for a short walk. Thirty minutes a day of walking is enough to boost your mood and reduce stress. In fact, any amount of exercise is a stress reducer. Don't skip it, unless the stress is physically restrictive in nature. At the very least, when facing long periods of work, take frequent breaks every hour. Stand up, stretch, and walk around a bit. Alternatively, when experiencing stress, take the opportunity to try out various alternative medicine and self-help therapies to help you relax and stay focused. Examples include hydrotherapy, guided meditation, controlled breathing, stretching or yoga, and therapeutic massage.

• **Don't be afraid to ask for help and support** – Discuss stress issues with your family. At the very least, stay in touch with people who can provide emotional and spiritual support during tough times. True friends and close family can give you an extra boost to handle upcoming stressful events or challenges. In contrast, being around toxic people can make you more susceptible to stress along with the associated negative influences. Be able to identify those people who are in need of dragging others, like you, down to their level. If you do not have to live or associate with such people, attempt to separate yourself from such relationships.

*   *   *

Optionally, consider keeping a journal to record and track regular stressors in your day-to-day life and how you deal with them. Use this journal every time you feel stressed. This process can not only help you identify when you are experiencing symptoms of stress, but it can also help you find more effective ways to prevent or cope with stress.

When it comes to managing stress, it is important to inform and educate yourself as much as possible on the subject and the sources so that you will be better prepared. It will also provide motivation to improve your mental state.

Unfortunately, stress is a risk factor that, despite its importance, is ignored by so many. In combination with other risk factors such as obesity, it can be even more deadly [101]. If left unchecked, stress can also lead to bad lifestyle choices, further compounding its negative effect on your long-term health as well as that of your family. Although much of the science behind stress reduction is unproven, the good news is that stress can be mitigated through common sense applications.

Do not allow stress to control you. Take action to control it. This is the common sense approach and smart way to achieve health and longevity.

Putting it all Together

We discussed the importance of sleep for long-term health. We looked at common sense actions to improve quality of sleep, which we found is as important as the amount of time we dedicate to rest.

We also discussed the role stress plays in health and how to address potential problems early. Along with other risk factors such as obesity and bad lifestyle choices, we found that stress can compound health problems even further.

Remember that sleep and stress are interrelated. Both can perpetuate a dangerous cycle of cause and effect. Stress can rob you of your sleep, and lack of sleep can raise your stress level, so it is important not to dismiss these problems as trivial. In most cases, they will not go away on their own.

Also, consider that lack of sleep and stress are risk factors that can be just as serious as any other life-altering medical conditions if they are allowed to continue. When common-sense applications fail, we should seek help when we need it.

The following action steps can be taken right away to improve your health.

ACTION STEPS

1. Be sure to get enough sleep. Aim for <u>at least 6.5 to 7.5 hours of sleep</u> each night. Additionally, try to <u>go to sleep and wake up at approximately the same time</u>.

2. Create an <u>optimal environment for sleep</u>. Pay attention to <u>sound</u>, <u>light</u>, and <u>temperature</u>. Make adjustments and <u>remove sources of disruption</u>.

3. <u>Eliminate the negative factors that sabotage sleep</u>. To help determine what they are, keep a <u>sleep diary or journal</u> to track naps and late-day activities, meals, and medications.

4. Learn to <u>recognize the signs of stress</u>. Doing so will enable you to be proactive and interrupt the pattern or behavior that is causing it.

Chapter 6: Environmental Chemical Hazards

Chemical Exposure and Health

Chemicals exist all around us. There are well over 100,000 chemicals produced around the world and many of these have not been adequately tested to determine their effects on health and the environment [102]. Of course, there are also many more chemicals that exist naturally. Avoiding all of them is impossible, but minimizing unnecessary exposure is critical to long-term health.

Most chemicals are relatively harmless, but, as we have learned in this book, excessive exposure to anything can wreak havoc on our bodies. It is often easy to spot immediate tissue damage or irritation from highly toxic chemicals. This is the obvious danger. On the other hand, if precautions are not taken, trace amounts of seemingly harmless chemicals, and even chemicals with low toxicity, can build up in our bodies over time with no indication of damage. They contribute to something called our chemical load, and after passing a certain threshold, they can overwhelm our natural ability to purge them effectively. From this point, later in life, the subtle effects of this increased chemical load may then manifest itself as chronic disease.

When it comes to long-term exposure to trace amounts of harmful chemicals of varying toxicity, the potential **health problems** are as follows.

● Chronic inflammation, as a result of excessive exposure to **toxic chemicals**, can potentially increase the risk of chronic diseases such as **heart disease**, **diabetes**, **Alzheimer's disease**, **stroke**, **arthritis**, and certain types of **cancer**.

• Chronic inflammation, as a result of **gradual buildup of trace chemicals** in our bodies, can increase our susceptibility to chronic diseases across-the-board.

• Long-term or excessive exposure to **air pollution** can increase our risk of **heart disease**, **stroke**, **chronic obstructive pulmonary disease** (lung disease), and **lung cancer** [103].

*   *   *

Air pollution in particular seems to be the hidden killer that doesn't get a lot of attention. The World Health Organization estimates that one in eight deaths worldwide is caused by such pollution [103]. With the greater variety of chemicals in the atmosphere and in our home, we need to pay more attention to them and their long-term effects on our health.

To reduce exposure to all chemicals, we have to be somewhat familiar with the sources. We'll start with household chemicals.

Household Chemicals

Chemicals improve the quality of our lives. As such, there are many different types of chemicals located throughout the home. Household chemicals include paint, cleaners, aerosol sprays, pesticides, deodorizers, and mothballs. Table 12 lists some of the common household chemicals and their locations [104, 105]. Notice that medicines are also classified as chemicals!

Many of these chemicals are used daily and are perceived to be harmless. However, if handled in an unsafe manner, even low toxicity chemicals have the potential to be dangerous to our long-term health. It is important to think about how often we use them and how often we ignore the risk.

Location	Household Chemicals
Basement	Paint; paint stripper and thinner; turpentine; stain; varnish
Bathroom	All-purpose cleaners; disinfectants (e.g. bleach); mold and mildew removers, drain cleaners, tub and tile cleaners; toilet bowl cleaners; window and glass cleaners; aerosol sprays
Bedroom	Mothballs
Garage	Antifreeze; motor oil; transmission fluid; windshield washer fluid; brake fluid; gasoline; car polish and wax; vehicle batteries
Kitchen	Dishwashing detergents; all-purpose cleaners; oven cleaners; disinfectants (e.g. bleach); air fresheners; window and glass cleaners; batteries; insect bait or traps
Living room	Carpet, rug, and upholstery cleaners; furniture polish; air fresheners; household foggers
Medicine Cabinet	Prescription medications; over-the-counter medications
Outdoor Shed	Pesticides; herbicides; fungicides; weed killer; fertilizer; insect repellants; swimming pool chemicals (e.g. chloride tablets)
Utility or Laundry Room	Laundry detergent; stain remover; fabric softeners; all-purpose cleaners; bleach; fluorescent light bulbs (if broken); insect repellents; pet flea and tick treatments

Table 12 – Location of common household chemicals. Many of these chemicals are used daily and are perceived to be harmless. Notice that medicines are also classified as chemicals.

The following common sense measures will help avoid excessive exposure to such chemicals.

• **Purchase the least toxic products** – Select the least toxic household products or find nontoxic alternatives. Pay attention to specific keywords on the product label such as **danger** or **poison** (most toxic), **warning** (moderately toxic), or **caution** (slightly toxic). For practical purposes, if there is no such label, the product is considered nontoxic [106].

• **Use less toxic homemade alternatives** – Consider using homemade versions of popular products in place of commercial products. For example, you can make your own deodorizer spray by combining a teaspoon of baking soda, a teaspoon of vinegar, and two cups of hot water in a spray bottle to remove odors. Additional examples are shown in table 13 [107, 108]. These products will almost always be less toxic than their store-bought counterparts. Other recipes for alternatives are widely available on the Internet. If you can't make your own, try using water-based products from the store. These will have a relatively lower concentration of chemicals due to dilution [109].

• **Don't stockpile** – This is probably the simplest way to reduce exposure. If you only buy what you need, when you need it, you decrease the risk of misuse or accidental release.

• **Follow directions carefully** – Use products only for their intended purposes and **use only the recommended concentration**. Using more of a product than directed does not necessarily translate to greater effectiveness. Furthermore, high concentrations may result in exposure that is beyond safe limits for regular use. Obviously, this is more difficult to keep track of if the label is removed. Be sure to contact the manufacturer if you have any questions regarding safe use.

• **Use products in well ventilated areas** – Use or apply in well ventilated areas or use outside. When indoors, turn on exhaust fans or open windows to vent chemical vapors outside.

Household Chemical	Homemade or Less Toxic Alternative
Air Freshener	Bowl of fragrant dried herbs or flowers
All-purpose Cleaner	Mixture of 1 cup vinegar; 1 cup water
Deodorizer Spray	Mixture of 1 tsp baking soda; 1 tsp vinegar or lemon juice; 2 cups hot water
Disinfectant	Mixture of 20 drops tea tree oil; 20 drops emulsifier (e.g. liquid soap); 1 cup water or vinegar
Fabric Softener	Ball of Aluminum foil
Floor Cleaner	Mixture of ¼ cup washing soda; 1 tbsp. liquid castile soap; ¼ cup vinegar; 8 liters hot water
Furniture Polish	Plain olive oil, almond, or walnut oil
Glass Cleaner	Mixture of ½ cup liquid castile soap; 3 tbsp. vinegar; 2 cups water
Tub and Tile Cleaner	Mixture of ¼ cup baking soda; ½ cup white vinegar
Upholstery Cleaner	Mixture of ½ cup liquid castile soap; 3 tbsp. water

Table 13 – Homemade alternatives to commercial household chemicals. These products will almost always be less toxic than their store-bought counterparts. Other recipes are widely available on the Internet.

● **Don't mix or burn** – Mixing chemicals can change their properties in a way that is not intended and the result may be a new mixture that is unsafe for household use. In particular, it can result in vapors that are toxic or flammable. Should containers be compromised by rust or damage, chemicals can combine to generate dangerous fumes and heat. This may be unrelated to long-term health, but it is important to point out that some common chemical mixtures can even cause fires from spontaneous combustion.

To reduce risk of any accidental occurrence, don't store incompatible products together. Make sure the caps are tightly sealed and secured. Likewise, don't burn plastics, paints, insulation, or anything that has the potential to release toxic fumes.

• **Store in safe place** – Keep products in their original containers and always follow instructions for proper storage. Elevate stored chemicals off of the floor or slab to avoid moisture, floods, and spills. Note that added moisture can deteriorate containers and distribute the contents locally or to other locations in the home or shop. It could also react with the chemical itself, creating a dangerous vapor.

As a rule, keep chemicals away from food storage and living areas. For example, keep food in the pantry, and move chemicals into a utility enclosure or some other isolated location. Food and chemicals do not belong together.

• **Dispose of chemicals correctly** – Follow directions on the container for disposal. Approved disposal methods may include rinsing, recycling, saving for toxic waste collection, flushing down the drain, or discarding in the trash [110]. Contact your local poison control center if you are not sure what to do. At the very least, if putting approved chemicals in the trash, try to wrap containers in a newspaper or bag before throwing them away to reduce the risk of human contact after discarding.

As a word of warning, **do not try to bury or dump hazardous substances in the ground**. Doing so could contaminate wells nearby, contaminate garden crops through runoff, or otherwise present a persistent health hazard before weathering can sufficiently break down the chemical.

• **Discard old medicines** – Medicines are chemicals too! Check the expiration date on both prescription and over-the-counter medications periodically. If they are old, discard them as instructed on the label.

• **Wash your hands more often** – After handling any chemical known to be toxic or otherwise, be sure to wash your hands with soap and water. Make this practice a habit. This is even more important when dealing with chemicals such as household pesticides, which are full of dangerous toxins. In some circumstances, high pesticide concentrations can make you deathly ill, so be sure not to touch your eyes, nose, mouth, or any other part of your body until your hands are thoroughly cleaned.

*   *   *

For more information on the safety of household chemical products, the U.S. Department of Health and Human Services has compiled a Household Products Database which details the health risks from handling and exposure. It is available on their website [111].

Building Materials and Furnishings

As a result of the use of certain building materials and furnishings, exposure to chemicals and other pollutants can be expected. And depending on the age of the home, this exposure may be unavoidable. Since we spend so much time in the home, we are in close proximity to these chemicals for long periods of time. Additionally, these materials can be a persistent source of air pollution that can reduce the air quality within the home. Whatever the circumstance, there are a few common sense measures that can be taken to minimize the risk associated with these sources [112].

● **Keep all surfaces free of dust** – Chemicals, such as lead, can accumulate as dust over time. To minimize exposure to these particles, keep the home clean by wiping down surfaces and vacuuming often. This will also reduce biological pollutants in the home substantially.

● **Repair damaged or deteriorating structures as soon as possible** – Materials that degrade over time will no longer be sealed and certain chemicals may become dangerous when exposed to air. As an example, in older homes and buildings, one of the more dangerous materials is asbestos. Asbestos can exist in floor tiles, walls, ceilings, insulation, roofing, and siding. Intact asbestos is not dangerous, but if it is disturbed and distributed in the air as dust particles, it is dangerous when inhaled. The only remedies for this are to seal and enclose the toxic material or replace it entirely.

• **Minimize exposure to formaldehyde and chemical treatments** – Formaldehyde sources include plywood, textiles, laminated furniture, cabinets, draperies, glues and adhesives, and foam insulation. This pollution is more common in new homes, and will emit less as the materials age. When it comes to new furniture, put newer products in well ventilated areas at first, especially if they have a strong chemical smell.

Ultimately, the best defense against any such chemical exposure is to maintain good airflow in the home.

• **Minimize lead exposure** – For older homes and buildings, lead could be a problem in both paint and plumbing. To reduce exposure, remove any lead based paint that is deteriorating. For lead pipes, run only cold water and seek an alternative source when drinking or preparing food. For all other cases, make sure to minimize dust accumulation on all surfaces.

• **Wash your hands** – Be sure to wash your hands often, especially before you eat. This is a good sanitary habit to have and will reduce trace exposure from contact with surfaces and other chemicals around the home.

Indoor Air Pollution

There are a number of factors that can contribute to poor air quality in the home including inadequate air circulation and the release of combustible by-products such as secondhand smoke, carbon monoxide, and nitrogen dioxide. Poor air circulation, for example, can lead to a more toxic atmosphere indoors, no matter how polluted the air is outside. Since we spend a lot of time inside the home, this exposure can be devastating over the long term.

Air pollution inside the house can be difficult to diagnose. Table 14 lists some of the signs that a potential problem exists in the home [113].

Unusual odors	Feeling healthier outside
Lack of ventilation indoors	Damaged pipes and chimneys
Noticeably stale and stuffy air	Unvented combustible appliances
Faulty climate control equipment	Unexplained irritation while indoors
Recent remodeling work	

Table 14 – Signs of increased exposure to indoor air pollutants. Air pollution inside the house can be difficult to diagnose.

To fix potential problems and prevent new ones, the following are some common sense guidelines for reducing exposure to indoor air pollutants.

• **Reduce exposure to secondhand tobacco smoke** – This is obvious. Smoking and prolonged exposure to second-hand smoke are both extremely dangerous to long-term health. Therefore, it is recommended that all smoking be done outdoors in an area where the smoke does not seep inside the house and affect otherwise healthy individuals.

• **Make sure combustible appliances are safe** – Make sure appliances such as gas ovens, stoves, water heaters, and other gas powered equipment are installed and vented properly. When in doubt about safety, install sensors around the home (e.g. carbon monoxide detectors). Alternatively, get these appliances checked by a qualified technician periodically. If installing combustible appliances, keep them as far away from living areas, such as bedrooms and living rooms, as possible. When able, install them in an isolated location, such as a utility room or basement, and make sure the areas are well-ventilated.

• **Make sure all ventilation systems are functioning properly** – Increasing ventilation and air exchange will reduce concentration of pollutants inside the house. Clean and inspect chimney, ducts, and pipes to ensure the system is properly functioning and sealed. Furthermore, make sure gas ranges and heaters are venting outdoors without obstruction. Also, don't forget about dryer ventilation in the utility room. Emissions from laundry products such as cleaners, air fresheners, and fragrances can significantly reduce indoor air quality [114].

• **Do not create additional sources of pollution** – Do not burn anything indoors unless it is in an approved appliance. Furthermore, do not leave cars, lawn mowers, or other equipment running when in the garage or when unattended.

• **Use indoor air cleaners** – Consider using ionizing purifiers or air filtration devices to help remove indoor air pollution. Note that these devices are only secondary control measures. The most effective way to minimize indoor air pollution is to reduce the sources of pollution and increase air flow throughout the home.

• **Use indoor house plants to clean the air** – Plants can absorb chemicals of all types, including formaldehyde, and transfer them to the soil where microorganisms break them down. The general recommendation is to use one potted plant per one hundred square feet [68].

• **Test your home for radon** – Radon is a naturally occurring radioactive gas in rocks and soil and therefore, is found just about everywhere. It seeps through openings in foundations, near sumps and drains, construction joints, and from the rock and soil surrounding the foundation. It is colorless, odorless, tasteless, and is the second leading cause of lung cancer in the United States [115]. Radon test kits are inexpensive and can be purchased at a hardware store or online. This testing should be done even if the structure was already built radon-resistant. In the event that radon levels are elevated, it is likely you will need professional services to correct the problem.

Outdoor Air Pollution

There are quite a few pollutants in the air outside our homes. The main culprits are ozone, particle pollution, carbon monoxide, nitrogen dioxide, and sulfur dioxide [116]. Table 15 lists some of the main sources of these pollutants.

Common Air Pollutants	Main Sources
Ozone	Industrial facilities; electric utilities; motor vehicles; gasoline vapors; chemicals
Particle pollution	Chemicals; soil particles; dust particles
Carbon monoxide	Combustible appliances (e.g. furnaces, gas stoves, wood fireplaces); motor vehicles
Nitrogen dioxide	Motor vehicles; power plants; lawn mowers; construction equipment
Sulfur dioxide	Power plants; industrial facilities; locomotives; construction equipment

Table 15 – Common air pollutants and their sources. We are undoubtedly exposed to many more unknown chemicals in the air.

Of course, in trace amounts, we are undoubtedly exposed to many more unknown chemicals in the air. The effects of a vast majority of these chemicals are largely unspecified. But, we do know that common pollutants such as ozone and particle pollution are increasing mortality and overall chronic disease risk worldwide.

To minimize exposure to the chemicals in the air outside the home, consider the following guidelines [68].

● **Keep your distance from sources of pollution** – It is not hard to deduce that air pollution is worse near sources of pollution. This means that, in general, it is best to stay as far away as possible from such sources, as the air will become progressively more contaminated and concentrated closer in. Use your common sense to avoid industrial and chemical storage areas.

● **Stay away from sources of smoke** – Anything that is burning or producing smoke will likely have enough heat to release and float toxic fumes and particles downwind. This can be said for something as simple as secondhand smoke from a cigarette. Also, stay indoors when there is smoke in the air from wood stoves, fireplaces, burning vegetation, or forest fires. If you are burning anything outdoors, make sure that people (and nearby living areas) are upwind of the smoke. Don't endanger the health of your neighbors and your friends.

● **Avoid outdoor activities when pollution level is higher** – Avoid ozone on smoggy days by staying indoors. Maximum concentrations typically occur in the afternoons on hot summer days. So, in the summer, plan outdoor activities in the morning. Note that on windy days, any specific type of particle pollution may be reduced in terms of volume (through dispersion); however, more of the particles will be released over a larger area.

The Environmental Protection Agency maintains an air quality rating system for the main air pollutants for larger cities in the United States [117]. So, if you are living in a major metropolitan area, you should pay attention to local alerts on television and radio, and spend less time outdoors when the risk level is moderate or higher.

● **Minimize exposure through behavior** – To avoid particle pollution, you should not linger around busy roads, rush hour thoroughfares, or near factory environments. These areas are filled with spilled chemicals and byproducts of toxic emissions. That also means jogging or doing yard work by busy roads is not advised. On hot smoggy days, it is safer to exercise indoors.

• **Create your own green belt** – A green belt is just an area of vegetation grown to make the air in the immediate vicinity cleaner. Consider this the next time you plan your landscape. Like a natural air filter, additional vegetation can absorb chemicals in the air and, depending on placement, can impede the movement of airborne particles. So, with enough density, vegetation can reduce exposure to chemicals around the outside of the home.

Water Pollution

When it comes to clean and safe water, we generally don't need to worry about municipal water supplies. Such systems have safeguards in place to detect, prevent, and remove chemical contamination of all types. If this source has not been seriously compromised in some way, the water can be considered safe to use. Even so, chorine and many other trace elements are not completely removed by the city system. So, in order to minimize exposure to these chemicals, and keep your pipes clean, it is recommended that you consider installing your own softening and filtration systems for water you drink and bath with.

If you are using well water or get your water from a private water supply, it may be a good idea to have it periodically tested for safety [118]. In reference to wells, groundwater can be contaminated from another point of entry (e.g. another well or landfill nearby). So, even if you are responsible with your water system, it can still be contaminated from sources outside your control.

Again, always keep in mind, just because you have access to a municipal water system, it does not mean you are risk-free when it comes to water pollution. There may be some level of contamination in water, no matter where it comes from [119]. For instance, toxic chemicals can still enter your system between the water supply and your home due to damaged plumbing. In this case, there may not be sufficient dilution of the chemical to guarantee good health. It is for this reason alone that you should consider testing your water periodically. Contact your local health department for further information on water testing services in your area.

Chemicals in the Garden

Since chemicals exist in the air, soil, and water, our garden crops are vulnerable if left exposed. Since we eat these crops, the same advice covered earlier in the book applies here, except that we are also responsible for growing the food. With this additional control, we have the added responsibility of ensuring that our own food is safe to eat after harvest.

Consider the following recommendations to keep chemicals out of your own food supply [68].

• **Don't garden near sources of pollution** – This includes places where chemicals are stored or are persistent. For example, you should never grow crops near roadsides. These areas introduce fumes as well as toxic particles that can be splashed or kicked up by passing cars. Furthermore, those same areas often have been exposed to chemicals such as pesticides. So, the farther you stay away from such sources, the better.

• **Pay attention to water runoff** – Rainwater runoff can carry pollutants from one location to another. Since low-lying or otherwise vulnerable crops will absorb the chemicals carried by this water, be sure to elevate garden plots or use vegetative barriers to prevent chemicals and other particles from entering your garden. This is especially important if your plants are downstream from a source of pollution. If you are in an urban area where you have less control over the environment, consider growing crops in containers. Container gardening gives you the greatest control over soil content and water.

• **Avoid pesticides and chemical fertilizers** – Try to find less toxic methods to control pests and enhance the growth of your garden. If, after exhausting nonchemical options, you need to resort to chemicals, use only what you need to correct your problem. For example, if you know what pest is affecting your crops, use a narrow-spectrum pesticide for that pest instead of a stronger broad-spectrum pesticide designed for a wide variety of pests. When it comes to using chemicals in your garden, be a minimalist.

• **Make use of additional vegetation** – Create a decorative and protective landscape around your garden crops. These extra plants will absorb and breakdown chemicals in the soil nearby, and will also prevent runoff from contaminating crops.

Putting in All Together

Although we are constantly surrounded by chemicals, we can take common sense steps to reduce unnecessary exposure to them. Naturally, highly toxic substances must be handled safely to prevent immediate injury and sickness. For substances with lower toxicity, the damage may not be apparent in the short term. But, it is important to remember that mishandling them can still cause harm as we age. Therefore, we must learn to respect all chemicals as potentially harmful and avoid unnecessary extremes that can lead to health complications in the long run.

As previously discussed, we can increase overall resiliency of our bodies to stressors of all types. By extension, this also means we can reduce our vulnerability to air pollution as well as other types of chemical exposure. So, no matter what environment we are in, the most effective way to counter ubiquitous chemical hazards is to eat a healthy diet, exercise regularly, and get plenty of sleep. Furthermore, a healthy lifestyle, along with common sense avoidance measures, will decrease our overall chemical load and reduce the risk of chronic disease across-the-board. As shown throughout this book, these approaches are amazingly simple.

The following action steps can be taken right away to improve your health.

ACTION STEPS

1.	To reduce exposure to household chemicals, <u>use the least toxic products</u>, <u>don't stockpile</u>, and always <u>follow the instructions</u> on safe use, storage, and disposal.
2.	To reduce concentration of air pollutants, <u>maintain good ventilation</u> and <u>adequate air flow</u> throughout the home.
3.	To limit sources of pollution, <u>keep your home well-maintained</u> and <u>clean</u>. Remove or replace deteriorating building materials as soon as possible. Make sure combustible appliances are installed properly and are in good working order.
4.	To increase resiliency to toxic chemicals in the atmosphere and in the home, be sure to <u>eat a healthy diet</u>, <u>exercise regularly</u>, and <u>get plenty of sleep</u>.

Chapter 7: Biological Pollutants and Germs

Biological Contamination in the Environment

We share the same space with numerous tiny biological organisms and substances, both inside and outside the home. Some of them are harmful, while others are not. And both can be considered a form of biological contamination. The ones that are harmful may only affect us in the short-term, manifesting as a common cold or temporary illness. Even if this is the case, a persistent unhealthy environment, populated by too many of these contaminates, can wreak havoc on our bodies if the exposure is excessive or occurs too often. That is why it is important to pay attention to our immediate environment, especially in places where we live or spend a lot of time.

Many of these biological organisms and substances are microscopic and are invisible to the naked eye. Because of this, we tend to ignore their existence and how they affect us. In the short term, we might stop to think about this when we catch the equivalent of a common cold or we have a minor allergic reaction. But, long-term affects should not be ignored, especially when there are so many easy things we can do to mitigate the health risks that are associated with them.

To begin, we can break down these potentially harmful organisms and substances into two main categories. One is called a biological pollutant. Biological pollutants are the source of common allergies that many of us suffer from. Examples include pollen, dust, animal dander, and mold. The other category is called a germ. A germ is a harmful microscopic organism, such as a bacteria or a virus, which can cause illness. Some germs result in an illness that is short-term in nature, while others can result in long-term chronic disease, which we certainly want to avoid.

When it comes to biological contamination in our environment, the potential **health problems** include the following.

• Chronic inflammation, as a result of exposure to **biological pollutants**, can potentially increase the risk of chronic diseases such as **heart disease**, **diabetes**, **Alzheimer's disease**, **stroke**, **arthritis**, and certain types of **cancer**.

• Excessive exposure to the same **biological pollutants** can increase susceptibility to other dangerous diseases, such as **asthma** [120].

• Chronic inflammation from excessive and high-frequency exposure to **germs** can increase the risk of chronic diseases such as **cancer** [121].

• Exposure to the wrong **germs** can result in early death, as in the case of **influenza and pneumonia**, or long-term infectious diseases, such as Tuberculosis.

• A **weakened immune system**, resulting from any of the above repeated illnesses, can increase the risk of chronic disease across-the-board.

*　　*　　*

Allergic reactions to biological pollutants are quite common. When we have an allergic reaction to something, our immune system goes into high gear to try to remove the foreign substance. Symptoms include watery, itchy eyes, wheezing, runny nose, congestion, coughing, headache, dizziness, and fatigue. Some individuals develop immunity to the substances commonly associated with these allergies. Others seem to suffer incessantly, and it can get worse with age. If something cannot be done about this hypersensitivity, the persistent inflammation can weaken our bodies and make us sick over time.

When it comes to germs, not all exposure is bad. To elaborate, when we were younger, it was the limited exposure to harmful microscopic organisms that helped us build a healthy immune system. So, even today, we should not be living in complete isolation. We actually need a certain amount of exposure to stay healthy. On the other hand, if we are constantly barraged by infections, this can be considered a chronic condition in its own right. At a certain point, further exposure, especially at high concentrations and longer durations, is pointless and does us more harm than good. We have to find a happy medium.

Unfortunately, no matter what we do, we cannot completely avoid biological pollutants and germs. We still have to go outside, breathe air, work with other people, touch all types of surfaces, and eat food. So, naturally, some exposure is assumed. To achieve moderation, the solution is simply to **live in a more sanitary environment** and **utilize common sense avoidance techniques**. Since we can't create a perfect environment anyway, this will keep exposure to a minimum, and more importantly, prevent infection from the extremely harmful germs that are out there.

This chapter will focus on common sense steps to reasonably deal with both biological pollutants and germs. We cannot protect ourselves from all of them of course, but the control measures listed herein will both **reduce the concentration** and **reduce the time of exposure**. This is all we need for our bodies to develop and maintain a healthy immune system while avoiding potential health problems associated with excessive exposure.

Common Biological Pollutants and Germs

As previously stated, biological pollutants are organisms and other substances that have the potential to cause allergic reactions. They are often referred to as allergens and can be found almost anywhere. Allergens can be absorbed through the skin and eyes, or inhaled through the nose or mouth.

Common types of biological pollutants (allergens) include the following [122].

● **Dust mites** – These small organisms are a component of house dust. Dust mites thrive in warm and damp environments. They can be found in mattresses, upholstery, curtains, carpets, and stuffed animals.

● **Mold and mildew** – Mold and mildew are fungi or fungi-like organisms. Both thrive in warm and damp environments. Inside the home, they can be found in bathrooms, kitchens, and utility rooms. Outside the home, they can be found on leaves and in standing water.

● **Pollen** – This substance is released by trees, weeds, and grasses. Pollen is a seasonal allergen. The pollen count for an area depends on time of year and geographic location. Information on pollen count is typically included in the local weather forecast.

● **Animal Dander** – This is a substance (a protein) that comes from animal skin, hair, and saliva. Cats are a significant source of this allergen.

● **Cockroaches** – These black or brown insects, their droppings, and leftover parts are common sources of allergies in the home.

● **Insects** – Common sources of insect allergies include the honey bee, yellow jacket, hornet, wasp, and fire ant. Venom, from stings, and contact with insects and insect parts can also cause an allergic reaction.

*   *   *

Obviously we cannot eliminate such biological pollutants, as they are ubiquitous in our environment. However, we can significantly reduce exposure by decreasing the concentration in our immediate area and avoiding contact.

*   *   *

Germs are also found everywhere in the environment. They can be absorbed through the skin and eyes, inhaled through the nose and mouth, or enter through a break in the skin, as in a cut or a scrape.

There are two main types of germs covered in this chapter: bacteria and viruses [123].

● **Bacteria** – Bacteria are single cell organisms that can live inside or outside of our bodies. Examples of diseases caused by bacteria include strep throat, tuberculosis, and urinary tract infections. Not all bacteria are harmful. For example, bacteria, called normal flora, live naturally in our bodies and aid in digestion. They also live in the air, soil, and water. They break down chemicals, decompose organic matter, and even play a part in the weather cycle. In essence, they are critical for life. However, sometimes, when bacteria enter our bodies, they cause disease. These harmful variants are the ones we are trying to avoid.

● **Viruses** – A virus is a very small particle that encapsulates genetic material (containing viral genes). Examples of diseases caused by viruses include the common cold, bronchitis, influenza, measles, and chickenpox.

*   *   *

As stated previously, there is no way to isolate ourselves from everyday germs. We cannot walk around with a biocontainment suit and a respirator, nor would we want to. The only way we can minimize exposure is to use this knowledge to our advantage. Doing so will ensure that the concentration of any germ is low enough to allow our immune system to neutralize the threat without an extreme inflammatory response.

Control Measures Inside and Outside the Home

There are a number of things we can do to reduce the concentration of biological pollutants and germs that are the cause of irritation and illness. The following control measures are designed to minimize exposure to one or more biological contaminates in a common sense fashion. They are organized into ten categories including dust control, moisture control inside, moisture control outside, air quality control inside, air quality control outside, animal control, pest control, cleaning, sanitizing, and personal hygiene (table 16).

Control Measures	Biological Pollutants						Germs	
	Dust Mites	Mold and Mildew	Pollen	Animal Dander	Cock-roach	Insects	Bacteria	Viruses
Dust Control	●	●	●	●	●	●		
Moisture Control – Inside	●	●						
Moisture Control – Outside		●				●		
Air Quality Control – Inside	●	●	●	●				
Air Quality Control – Outside			●					
Animal Control				●				
Pest Control					●	●		
Cleaning	●	●	●	●	●	●		
Sanitizing							●	●
Personal Hygiene	●	●	●	●	●	●	●	●

Table 16 – Overview of control measures for several types of biological pollutants and germs. The control measures are organized into ten categories including dust control, moisture control inside, moisture control outside, air quality control inside, air quality control outside, animal control, pest control, cleaning, sanitizing, and personal hygiene.

Dust Control:

By limiting contact with dust particles, you can reduce exposure to biological pollutants such as **dust mites**, **mold and mildew**, **pollen**, **animal dander**, **cockroaches**, and **insect parts** [122, 124]. To a limited extent, controlling dust can also help reduce the concentration of germs.

• **Keep all surfaces free of dust** – Keep living and work areas as clean as possible. Use dusters, microfiber cloths, dry sweepers, and floor cleaners to remove as much dust off exposed surfaces as possible. The use of a wet mop or dampened cloth will keep dust from being kicked up while cleaning. Also, by removing items off of the floor and decluttering in general, you will be able to clean more thoroughly. Try to do this at least once a week. Don't forget to clean venetian-style blinds, which are commonly overlooked.

• **Wash bedding regularly** – Clean sheets, blankets, comforters, and other bedding weekly, preferably using warm or hot water.

• **Vacuum regularly** – Vacuum carpets and upholstery using a vacuum cleaner with a high-efficiency particulate air filter (HEPA). These filters will trap the vast majority of any tiny particles picked up by the vacuum cleaner. Also consider the use of a water-based vacuum cleaner, if you can afford one, to trap contaminates more effectively.

• **Avoid using dust-gathering materials** – Avoid using bedroom carpets and floor rugs, which can both trap dust particles easily and can be difficult to clean. Also, avoid upholstered furniture, especially in the bedroom. At the very least, use slipcovers to make cleaning easier. Consider the same advice in other living areas where you spend a lot of time. Avoid using heavy curtains in the home. These are all ideal habitats for allergens.

• **Use allergen impermeable materials** – Allergen impermeable materials should be used to cover mattresses, box springs, and all pillows. Dust mites that get inside the material will linger and multiply.

• **Wash or remove stuffed animals** – Stuffed animals are another ideal habitat for dust mites and can accumulate animal dander and other allergens. If you can't realistically get rid of them when they are dirty, try washing them thoroughly in hot water. An alternative is to put them in a freezer bag and keep them in a freezer overnight. This will effectively kill the dust mites, but will not remove the allergens (e.g. insect parts and animal dander). To deal with the remnants, you will need to wash them afterwards.

Moisture Control – Inside:

By reducing the moisture level indoors, you reduce exposure to biological pollutants such as **mold and mildew**, as well as **dust mites**. For mold in particular, a persistent moisture problem will cause the infestation to come back no matter how many times you clean and kill the mold. You have to address this problem at the source [112, 125].

• **Keep surfaces mostly free of mold and mildew** – Clean surfaces with a mold and mildew remover, disinfectant, or antibacterial cleaner. Consider the application of a steam cleaner, which is extremely effective. Be sure to clean shower walls, bathtubs, sinks, ceiling tiles, and wallboards. Don't forget to clean crevices where the floor meets the tub or shower. Also clean areas under the sink and near window frames and sills. Note that you must control relative humidity to stop the mold and mildew from reappearing.

• **Lower the relative indoor humidity** – Relative humidity should be maintained between 30 and 50 percent. This can be measured with a hygrometer, perhaps included in your climate control system. Otherwise, you can purchase one for less than ten dollars. Use dehumidifiers to lower humidity levels anytime and air conditioners to lower humidity levels during summer months.

• **Remove any problem sources of excess moisture** – Fix existing water problems in the house. Whether they are leaks or condensation issues, not doing so will make control over moisture and humidity levels an uphill battle. This is another reason to fix leaky roofs, doors and windows as soon as possible.

• **Improve ventilation** – Use or install exhaust fans to vent air from places such as the kitchen and bathroom where there are persistent water sources. Also, make sure attics and crawl spaces are well-ventilated by using soffit and roof vents as needed.

• **Remove materials that encourage mold and mildew growth** – To reduce the impact of existing high-moisture environments, consider replacing or removing all carpets. Opt for wood or vinyl flooring instead.

• **Don't make the problem worse** – Don't use basements as living areas unless you can ensure they stay ventilated and dry. Note that any moisture entering through masonry walls or floors has to be addressed and contained. Limit use of humidifiers in the home and limit the number of indoor houseplants to one per room. With that said, keep in mind that plants are beneficial in that they can filter other types of contaminates in the air.

Moisture Control – Outside:

A high moisture level outdoors will create numerous tiny habitats for biological pollutants and other pests near your home. By reducing the moisture level, you reduce exposure to allergens such as **mold and mildew**, as well as reduce the **insect** population [68].

• **Keep standing rain water around the house to a minimum** – After a rainfall, empty the water from containers, barrels, and tires in close proximity to the house. Also, keep the grass cut and the landscape maintained so that rainwater will evaporate faster.

• **Reduce moisture level around the landscape** – If you garden or do landscaping, consider using drip irrigation to keep plants relatively dry (for less mold and mildew). Also, keep sufficient spacing between plants and shrubs to maintain good air flow between them.

• **Fix drainage issues around the house as soon as possible** – Drainage can be a complex topic on its own. However, there are a few common sense methods that can reduce the severity of drainage problems and prevent the accumulation of water. For example, use gutter extensions to direct flow of rain water away from the house. For walkways and developed areas that collect water, use porous bricks and tiles to allow for faster drainage. Other methods are costlier in terms of time and money, but you can plant more cover crops and shrubs around your landscape to accelerate drainage naturally. The roots of these plants create inlets into the ground for water to drain and give the soil more structure as well. The deeper the roots penetrate into the ground, the better the drainage potential. Other options include drainage ditches, perforated pipes, and ground elevation, but these solutions are more involved and the need for such remedies may indicate a more serious drainage issue.

• **Control the spread of mold and mildew** – Periodically clean mold and mildew around the outside of the house by using a cleaning solution (e.g. oxygen bleach), brushes, and a pressure washer or sprayer, depending on the surface. Serious mold and mildew problems may require professional cleaning services.

Air Quality Control – Inside:

By maintaining good air quality inside the house, you reduce exposure to airborne biological pollutants such as **dust mites**, **mold and mildew**, **pollen**, and **animal dander** [122].

• **Keep indoor air clean** – Change filters in your climate control system, which includes the heater and air conditioner, at least monthly. Consider using indoor air filters and ionizing purifiers to reduce the concentration of airborne particles in living areas.

• **Maintain adequate ventilation** – Use exhaust fans or a central air system to vent air regularly. Strangely enough, when ventilation in a house, especially a new one, is poor, the inside can quickly become more contaminated than the outside environment. So, ventilation is important to keep the numbers of airborne biological contaminates down overall. Don't forget about attics and crawl spaces either; they should be well-ventilated as well.

• **Don't make the problem worse** – Keep windows closed during days with a high pollen count.

Air Quality Control – Outside:

Obviously, we have very limited control over air quality outside our home. But, we also don't have to make the situation worse when we do go outside. Common sense avoidance will minimize exposure to allergens such as **pollen**.

• **Protect the mouth and eyes when doing work outside** – Use a mask, along with eye protection (e.g. safety glasses or goggles), when doing outside work such as mowing the lawn or using trimmers or blowers. This is especially important when there is a higher concentration of particles in the air. On windy days, it seems to be worse. Be sure to keep people with severe allergies inside with the windows closed until you are finished.

• **Avoid outdoor activities when the pollen count is high** – Allergy and pollen forecast information for your area is often available through local and national weather stations. If it is high, and you are vulnerable to the effects of pollen, you need to stay indoors to minimize exposure.

Animal Control Measures

Unfortunately, pets carry around many irritants, including **animal dander**. To minimize exposure to this protein and other substances, consider the following remedies.

• **Keep certain areas off limits to pets** – Use a child barrier or close the door to bedrooms. Pets should not be allowed in the bedroom, or on the bed for that matter. Once dander is present, **it can persist for up to six months** [122]. Consider doing the same for other sanitary living environments where you want to minimize exposure. Additionally, try to keep outdoor pets outside to keep them from tracking other contaminates into the home.

● **Keep your pets clean** – Shampoo pets once a week. This is obvious.

● **Don't forget to wash your hands after handling pets** – Wash hands with soap and water immediately after handling pets or animals. Do not touch your face, eyes, or nose unless your hands are thoroughly cleaned.

Pest Control Measures

Pest control is another complex topic, especially as it applies to gardening or landscaping. But, to control allergies triggered by pests, we only need to do enough to keep the general population of pests to a minimum. So, to minimize exposure to **cockroaches**, **insects**, and insect parts, consider the following common sense remedies in and around the house [68].

● **Maintain a buffer zone** – Consider setting up and maintaining a buffer zone around your home. The buffer zone is a clean area devoid of all plants, landscape trimmings, garden crops, compost piles, debris, garbage, wood piles, and anything else that can serve as a potential source for pests. Such sources should be located away from the house.

● **Secure sources of food** – Use sealed metal, glass, or heavy plastic containers to store your food, including pet food. Vulnerable containers made out of paper, cardboard, or thin plastic will not provide much protection from pests such as rodents. Once rodents gain access to the food, so do insects. So, consider placing flimsy storage containers within a large stronger container, like a heavy plastic bucket or metal garbage can. Also, make sure your garbage is sealed and the area around it is clean.

● **Pest proof your home** – Look for structural gaps and holes where insects and other pests can enter. Check both inside and outside your home. Potential entry points include cracks in brick mortar joints, areas around electric conduits and outlets, water and gas pipes, floor plumbing including tub inspection vents, doors, attic hatches, air intake and exhaust vents, soffit vents, fireplace and chimney openings, windows, back of cupboards, between floorboards, and floor molding. Once found, seal them with pest-resistant materials like metal sheets, caulking, joint compound, expanding foam, or mortar. When it comes to regular maintenance, previously applied sealing materials need to be checked periodically and reapplied as necessary.

● **Use pesticides** – Chemical pest control products come in spay, dust, or bait form. Consider periodically applying such products in and around the house to keep the population of insects and other pests down. It is good practice to avoid using broad-spectrum versions if possible. These are designed to kill a wide range of pests. So, if you can target a troublesome pest, such as the cockroach for example, select the appropriate pesticide that targets that particular pest. By using narrow-spectrum chemicals, you can avoid increasing the natural resistance of other troublesome species of insects in the process.

● **Protect yourself from stinging and biting insects** – Wear light-colored clothes when spending time outside. Certain insects are attracted to dark colors and dark spaces. Avoid lotions and perfumes, which can attract insects as well. Use insect repellants and place such products near the door to the outside as a reminder to use it. Don't forget to wear gloves and use repellant when working outside. And always increase your awareness of insects such as fire ants which are present above and below ground.

Cleaning and Sanitizing:

Cleaning involves removing dirt and grime from floors and surfaces. It is effective in reducing the population of **dust mites**, **mold and mildew**, **pollen**, **animal dander**, **cockroaches**, and **insects**.

Cleaning is typically done with regular soap and warm water. Note that it is not the same as sanitizing. Sanitizing will kill germs, including bacteria and viruses, whereas cleaning alone will not. However, you do have to clean first before you are able to sanitize a surface effectively. So, in that sense, keeping a home clean is absolutely critical to minimizing exposure to any biological pollutant or germ.

Good sanitary practices are the key to minimizing exposure to germs, such as **bacteria** and **viruses**, which are present on various surfaces. Use your favorite household cleaners, but keep in mind that the best disinfectant is a diluted bleach solution.

Consider the following guidelines for minimizing contact with both biological pollutants and germs in the home [126].

• **Clean and sanitize frequently touched objects** – Routinely clean and sanitize frequently touched objects such as doorknobs, faucets, handles, keyboards, peripheral devices, phones, cell phones, and other electronic devices.

• **Clean and sanitize frequently touched surfaces** – Be sure to routinely clean and sanitize all frequently touched surfaces such as tables, desks, and countertops. Note that germs such as viruses can remain viable on such surfaces for many hours.

• **Clean and sanitize the primary sources of germs** – Both the bathroom and kitchen provide warm, damp areas for germs to proliferate. In the bathroom, be sure to thoroughly clean and sanitize the toilet bowl, sink, faucet, and shower area, including tiled walls as well as the shower curtain. Do this regularly. In the kitchen, clean the countertops, walls, shelves, and cabinets, including the top of the cabinets, periodically. Regularly clean and sanitize all kitchen appliances. The use of steam cleaners can be very effective.

*   *   *

Note that if you spend a lot of time in certain public areas, such as an office or hospital environment, you may consider using disinfecting wipes to periodically sanitize objects and surfaces that you make contact with frequently.

Personal Hygiene:

By using good personal hygiene, you minimize exposure to biological pollutants and germs across the board, including **dust mites**, **mold and mildew**, **pollen**, **animal dander**, **cockroaches**, **insects**, **bacteria**, and **viruses**. Good personal hygiene is, in many ways, a universal control measure for our bodies. Consider the following recommendations [127].

• **Wash your hands with soap and water regularly** – One of the simplest ways to minimize body absorption of biological pollutants and germs is to wash your hands. Do it often. Table 17 brings to your attention some of the situations that require hand washing in order to minimize your own risk of illness, as well as risk to others.

When washing your hands, you should use soap and water. It is not necessary for the water to be warm or hot. The temperature will not be high enough to kill germs. However, the cleaning should be thorough. After applying soap, wash your hands in water **for at least 20 seconds**, rubbing your hands together vigorously to remove all particles and dirt. When soap and water is not available, you can resort to using a hand sanitizer. However, do not rely on hand sanitizers as your primary cleaning method.

Before	When to Wash Hands	After
●	Caring for sick individuals	●
●	Treating a cut or wound	●
	Using the toilet	●
	Using a public restroom	●
	Changing diapers	●
	Coughing, sneezing, or blowing nose	●
	Touching an animal	●
	In contact with animal feed or feces	●
	Handling pet food or pet treats	●
	Touching garbage or any other waste	●
	Using public exercise equipment	●
●	Preparing Food	●
●	Eating	
	Doing work outside	●
●	Gardening	●

Table 17 – When you should wash your hands. Some situations require hand washing before and after in order to minimize your own risk of illness, as well as risk to others.

● **Wash your hands defensively** – When washing hands in a public area such as restroom, it is worth taking a little extra care not to make contact with contaminated surfaces. Table 18 shows how this might be done. Note that you **should not touch the faucet handle** or **any part of the door** after you have washed your hands. Use a paper towel as indicated, or find an alternative means of avoiding contact.

How to Wash Hands Defensively	
1	Wet hands and let water run
2	Apply soap
3	Wash hands thoroughly
4	Rinse and let water run
5	Dry hands with paper towel
6	Do not throw towel away
7	Use towel to turn off water
8	Use towel to open the door
9	Throw towel away

Table 18 – Process for washing your hands defensively. In public areas, such as a restroom, you should not touch the faucet handle or any part of the door after you have washed your hands. Also, you should not touch your eyes, nose, or mouth before you have thoroughly cleaned your hands.

Also, you **should not touch your eyes, nose, or mouth** before you have thoroughly cleaned your hands.

If a public restroom has a hand dryer in lieu of towels, do not assume it is safe [128]. Unless the filter is changed, or cleaned and disinfected, consider it a source of blowing contaminates that have accumulated over time from the restroom environment.

● **Bathe more often** – Washing the entire body regularly with soap and water removes both biological pollutants and germs of all types from the surface of skin.

● **Wash your clothes more often** – Damp, sweaty, and dirty clothes are also perfect environments for allergens and germs. The fibers in clothing will trap dust, mold, animal dander, germs, and other substances.

● **Wear protective clothing when working in unsanitary environments** – For example, when cleaning surfaces that are possibly contaminated, consider wearing a facemask, eye protection, and gloves to avoid skin contact and splatter. When vacuuming or kicking up dust, wear a dust or allergy mask.

When All Else Fails

If you are having a hard time controlling biological pollutants in and around your home, all is not lost. You can acquire over-the-counter allergy medications (e.g. antihistamines), which will lessen the inflammatory response to allergens you are exposed to. However, every drug has side effects and such medication should only be considered as a temporary solution, not to be relied upon long-term if you can help it.

To get to the root of the problem, you must remove the allergen, remove the source of the allergen, or you must find a way to avoid it all together. Any other solution should probably be considered counterproductive, especially if the problem could have been remediated through common sense actions as discussed in this chapter. However, if the problem cannot be handled in this manner, there are some medical treatments, such as allergy shots or prescription drugs, which might lessen the symptoms. Still, they do not solve the original problem and therefore should be considered as a last resort.

In reference to germs such as bacteria and viruses, if you become infected, your immune system in most cases will neutralize the invading germ. You can use over-the-counter medications to ease the symptoms, and in some cases treat minor infections. However, it is largely your immune system that will do the heavy lifting.

Regarding bacterial infections, antibiotics are commonly used as a quick solution. Sometimes they are necessary for serious infections, but at other times, it seems that it is a matter of convenience to treat the infection fast and be done with it. Unfortunately, this persistent use of antibiotics can cause harmful side effects and may weaken your immune system in the long run. For example, antibiotics can indiscriminately kill good and bad bacteria in our bodies. Good bacteria, also referred to as normal flora, contribute to overall health and help to prevent the spread of harmful bacteria. When we use antibiotics to treat every minor infection, we reduce the population of good bacteria and this may make us more vulnerable to other diseases. This is why antibiotics should only be used as a last resort.

It is also important to remember, that whenever you do have to take antibiotics, you must use the whole dosage that was prescribed. You must not leave some of the antibiotics for later, and you should never give them to someone else. When using antibiotics, the symptoms may disappear and you may be tempted to throw the rest away. However, the remnants of bad bacteria may still be alive within you and may still reproduce. This condition could eventually lead to antibiotic-resistance, which is when the surviving bacteria become more resilient to the current antibiotics you are taking. And when future illnesses occur, that same antibiotic may no longer be effective.

Note that even vaccines for preventing viral infections are sometimes not as effective as one would hope. For example, recent flu vaccinations sometimes offer little protection when new variants of the virus appear. In short, you need to focus, now more than ever, on staying healthy and avoiding infection on your own. It is best not to depend on society to provide quick-fix medical solutions.

Remember that maintaining a healthy diet, staying physically active, and getting quality sleep all boost your immune system and make your body more resilient to infection and disease. This is the ultimate insurance against both biological pollutants and germs of all types. Also, these habits will make it easier to recover from illness when it inevitably occurs.

Naturally, you can rely on medical treatments as a backup for a serious illness.

Sexually Transmitted Infections and Long-Term Health

Although sexually transmitted infections and diseases were not discussed earlier in this chapter, it is important, now, to briefly mention how they affect long-term health. Some of these infections can be considered chronic diseases (e.g. HIV), while others are seemingly minor nuisances. Even if an infection produces no obvious symptoms, it can still weaken the immune system over time. The hidden nature of these diseases highlights how bacterial and viral infections can linger on (for months or years) with little to no warning of our current state. Often, we will not even realize the damage that is being done. And, whether we know about it or not, many of these infections have been linked to chronic diseases of all types [129] .

Sexually transmitted infections are unique in that all it takes to largely avoid them is a change in behavior. However, that has not stopped the increase in transmission rate around the world [129]. With such a widespread occurrence (more than one million new cases every day worldwide), we cannot predict or choose which ones we will be exposed to. The bottom line is that we cannot ignore the role of such infections in our long-term health, for it is not just a temporary problem. We should, at the very least, take basic precautions and act responsibly. If we don't, we risk much more later on when we are battling age-related chronic diseases and conditions.

Putting it All Together

In this chapter, we have covered how to deal with various types of biological pollutants and germs. Exposure is largely unavoidable, as many of them are ubiquitous in our environment. Plus, some exposure can be beneficial as long as it is moderated in terms of concentration and duration. However, if one continues to live in an unclean and unsanitary environment, exposure can increase to a level that is dangerous.

The objective of this chapter is to find a happy medium. This involves taking common sense steps to reduce exposure while not trying to live in isolation. By doing this, we allow our immune system to grow stronger, all the while reducing the risk of serious illness and chronic disease in the future.

Chapter 7: Biological Pollutants and Germs

The following action steps can be taken right away to improve your health.

ACTION STEPS

1. To reduce exposure to common biological pollutants, <u>keep living areas clean and dust-free</u>.

2. Address biological contamination problems at the source. For mold and mildew, cleaning is not enough. You must <u>lower relative indoor humidity</u> and <u>remove sources of excess moisture</u>.

3. Be sure to maintain good air quality in the home with <u>adequate ventilation</u> and <u>clean air filtration</u>.

4. Regularly <u>clean and sanitize frequently-touched surfaces</u> that accumulate germs, as well as areas that are the <u>primary source of germs</u>, such as bathrooms and kitchens.

5. <u>Wash your hands with soap and water</u>. Do it often. If your hands are contaminated, <u>don't touch your eyes, nose, or mouth</u> before you have thoroughly cleaned and sanitized them.

Chapter 8: Technology Related Health Hazards

The Potential Dangers of Modern Technology

Technology is all around us. From cell phones, mobile devices, computers, televisions, smart vehicles, and smart utilities, the list seems endless. Without a doubt, such modern technology is affecting our lifestyles in ways never seen before. The same can be said when it comes to how it affects long-term health.

The problem with all this technology is that it is being developed so fast that we can hardly keep up with the changes. Every year, a number of new gadgets and appliances are released on the market with astonishing regularity. Since short-term health effects are normally tested before release, as required by regulatory agencies, new technology is generally considered safe.

However, what about the long-term effects? It is the long-term health consequences that take years of research to ascertain. In the meantime, we spend more and more time using and living among this technology while oblivious to its potential health threats.

This chapter will focus, briefly, on some of the more subtle health risks that modern technology poses, particularly with respect to electronic devices and computers. Since we know dangerously little about how these devices affect us in the long-term, our recommendations are motivated by the need to take a precautionary approach, not to avoid using them altogether.

Unlike other topics, this type of risk is new and undefined because the research in these matters, while ongoing as we speak, is still inconclusive.

Therefore, it is not possible for us to fully define such risk. However, if taking certain precautions is of low-cost to the consumer in terms of time, money, and convenience, then it is realistic to recommend certain actions to minimize exposure or, at the very least, reduce the perceived adverse effects.

Simply stated, it is recommended that everyone consider a precautionary approach when it comes to enjoying the comforts of new technology until further research is conducted, or ultimately until it is demonstrated safe in the long-term.

The potential **health dangers** associated with **modern technology** include the following.

• **Long-term exposure to electromagnetic fields** (EMF) can lead to a variety of health problems, including an **increased risk** of various forms of **cancer** [130].

• **Long-term application of electronic devices and equipment** can lead to a variety of occupational disabilities, including **back and spine problems**.

• An **inactive lifestyle**, as encouraged by a high-tech work culture, can result in an **increased risk** of **obesity, high blood pressure, type 2 diabetes**, **heart disease, stroke, respiratory problems, cancer, osteoporosis, arthritis, sleep disorders**, and **mental health problems** [5, 6].

*   *   *

We begin by addressing the potential hidden dangers brought on by persistent electromagnetic fields.

Effects of Radiation from Electromagnetic Fields

Electromagnetic fields exist all around us. They are invisible to the naked eye and are mostly harmless [131]. Electromagnetic fields are generated from man-made sources such as electrical and electronic devices, and are used in power, industrial, communication, and personal electronics applications. These emissions, typically referred to as radio frequency (RF) radiation, are propagated through the atmosphere, carrying voice and data transmissions to locations across the globe.

In technical terms, a traveling electromagnetic field (EMF) consists of both electric and magnetic fields in motion at the same time. Electric fields are created by differences in voltage whereas magnetic fields are created by an electric current through a conductor. When a human is in the way of these moving fields, the result can be hazardous to health when, at any corresponding frequency, the absorbed energy of the waveform is strong enough.

There are two potential adverse consequences associated with exposure to EMF radiation [132]. The first is a non-ionizing effect from sources such as cell phone towers, power lines, and large radio antennas. The risk is the potential thermal damage to human tissue (e.g. a burn) if an individual touches an active transmitting antenna or is in close proximity to it for a certain amount of time. For the vast majority of people, this risk is largely irrelevant, since most of us do not work or otherwise loiter around such high-powered equipment.

The other effect is the alteration of cellular material and DNA from the ionizing capability of radiation, even at low power levels. This effect concerns us the most since it lacks sufficient scientific evidence to quantify damage to humans. Even though cellular damage is not as apparent to the public as thermal damage, we should still be aware of the possibility that it may, in a subtle fashion, be affecting the cells in our bodies and in our brains.

So, consider, for example, low-level electromagnetic fields such as those emitted by cell phones and small electronic Wi-Fi devices. These devices, as many now fear, have the potential to cause unexplained long-term health problems. In order for a device like this to transmit information, it must release radiation, often in the same frequency region as your microwave oven (table 19) [133]. This radiation is emitted during any voice or data communication, and even when a device is periodically communicating with a cell tower or wireless router on its own.

	RADIATION	SOURCES
HIGH FREQUENCY	**GAMMA**	Medical imaging
	X-RAY	Medical imaging, airport scanner
	ULTRAVIOLET	Sunlight
	VISIBLE LIGHT	Light bulb
	INFRARED	Television remote
	MICROWAVE	Cell phones, Wi-Fi, microwave oven
LOW FREQUENCY	**RADIO**	Broadcast television, AM/FM radio stations

Table 19 – An overview of the electromagnetic spectrum along with examples of sources of radiation. Notice that cell phones and Wi-Fi devices share the same frequency region as microwave ovens.

For a long time now, most of us have been using these small transmitting electrical devices. The same devices are often positioned close to us, sometimes resting on our skin or up against our bodies as wearable electronic devices. This trend will likely continue and, indeed, accelerate as technology expands.

It is the long-term cumulative effects on human tissue, and in particular our cells and DNA, that need more scientific investigation. This is an issue that the Federal Communications Commission has even acknowledged.

Not surprisingly, there have been recurring global complaints of headaches, memory loss, or even seizures from constant use of, or close proximity to, a cell phone or persistent wireless device (e.g. a home electric power meter installed as a smart meter). Even more disconcerting is the possibility that, for some of us, damage may be hidden for years to come. It may only surface after decades of exposure in the form of cancer or some other chronic disease.

Although the implications for related chronic diseases are largely unknown at this point, we can only surmise that low-level RF radiation (also known as electro-pollution) affects the body in some undefined manner. Since we are all using our devices a lot longer these days, it is entirely possible that some of us may eventually experience some degree of electronic sensitivity.

As indicated on their website, the Food and Drug Administration believe that there is no scientific evidence, up to now, that proves the link between RF exposure, from cell phones for example, and chronic disease. Definitive studies will take a while to conclude, since human tests are difficult to do over such a long time period and the effects are difficult to measure anyway. However, they acknowledge that **more research is needed**. In particular, there needs to be more studies on long-term exposure and effects, especially in developing children. Even the World Health Organization lists RF radiation as **possibly carcinogenic to humans**. And now, there are several significant large-scale studies currently being conducted on the issue [134]. Hopefully, we'll have the results soon.

The bottom line is: the **closer one is to a transmitting source** and the **longer one is exposed to such a source**, the **more serious the perceived potential damage is over the long term**. As of yet, there is still no definitive way to measure this damage. However, it is safe to conclude that something beyond our comprehension may be going on.

How to Reduce EMF Exposure

The number of sources of EMF radiation has increased dramatically over the years. Some operate very close to us, in some cases, for hours, or all day long as we work. Although the receiving portion of any communication has no adverse effects on the human cell or the DNA, most equipment must emit energy by transmitting when two-way communication is required. Note that even if you are not actively using your mobile phone for voice or data communication, your phone is still transmitting intermittently.

Consider the following transmitting sources when evaluating the individual or cumulative effect on long-term health. Note that in most cases, the transmitting lines to antennas are shielded and pose no hazard to health.

• Electrical power lines (especially high voltage lines overhead where you live or work)

• Microwave ovens (considered insulated high-powered devices but with some allowable leakage through the front panel)

• Radio towers and cell towers (hundreds of thousands in the U.S. alone)

• Amateur radio antennas (most operate at low power levels and at lower frequencies)

• Wireless access points (also referred to as wireless modems or wireless routers in your home or office)

• AM and FM broadcast radio stations

• Cell phones and smart phones

• Wearable electronics such as smart watches

• Satellite transmitting equipment (considered low power)

• Computer Wi-Fi network cards

• Any electronic device with a Wi-Fi connection, such as wireless cameras and baby monitors

• Smart meters (replacing analogue electric utility meters nationwide)

• Tablets, laptop computers, and e-readers

• Car, aircraft, and other vehicle electronic systems

• Police, fire, and other emergency communication devices

*　　　*　　　*

This list covers the more common sources. In the near future, we could see a dramatic expansion of this list. For example, plans are already underway to make most appliances in your home communicate wirelessly with each other and with an outside smart meter.

We cannot eliminate the hazard of environmental EMF exposure and most of it is harmless anyway. However, we can reduce exposure to radiation, including harmful radiation, by staying **as far away as possible from the source** (e.g. antenna) and, specifically, **away from the path or direction of maximum power**. Antennas within many devices, such as cell phones, are omnidirectional, meaning they transmit in all directions. Others are unidirectional (e.g. microwave dish) or bidirectional meaning they concentrate most power in one or two directions to increase signal strength. It is important to note that the power output from most antennas decreases very quickly as you move away from the antenna.

It is in our best interest to take precautionary actions due to the amount of time we spend using and interacting with these transmitting devices. The following low-cost remedies are some easy ways to minimize exposure, pending more research.

• **Go hands-free when transmitting voice** – Use a hands-free cell phone kit, or headset, when transmitting voice [135]. These kits use Bluetooth technology, which has a substantially weaker signal than a typical cell phone or smart device. With the short transmission distance of Bluetooth (e.g. only a few feet), the main transmitting device, such as a cell phone, can be held away from your head. Alternatively, you can use the speakerphone feature to accomplish the same thing. For many people, this is more convenient, and safer, then holding a phone in your hand all the time.

• **Do not sleep near sources of EMF** – Do not sleep with a mobile device in bed, especially near your head. Also, do not sleep immediately next to a wireless access point or a smart meter, which tracks household power consumption and regularly transmits the data. Look for this source outside the home, possibly on the other side of a bedroom wall. Note that radiation travels through walls and windows. Too short of a distance between the device and your head may eventually cause unexplained health complications and possibly affect sleep.

• **Carry mobile devices away from the body** – Avoid placing mobile devices in a pocket close to your skin or other sensitive areas, especially the heart and groin. Use body-worn accessories, such as a belt clip or holster. This type of accessory should keep the device a little farther away from the user, with enough distance to significantly reduce transmission exposure. Remember, mobile devices can still awaken and transmit on their own while not in use. Note that the Food and Drug Administration does not recommend using cell phone shield accessories to block radiation [135]. They may not work as advertised and may also interfere with operation of a device.

• **Reduce exposure to higher power equipment** – If you work near radio equipment (e.g. amateur and marine radio operations), work away from the higher power density lobes, or in the opposite direction of transmission for antennas that are directional. As a radio operator, reduce potential exposure by moving the antenna away from living areas and reduce the power to only what is needed to function.

• **Limit time of exposure** – You may consider limiting cell phone use to certain times of the day or for a predetermined amount of time. This has an additional benefit in that you may become more productive at work and at school. You may also consider turning off cell phones and other wireless devices when not in use, or turning off the wireless function while leaving the device on.

• **Don't rely exclusively on wireless technology** – If you have access to a landline phone system, use that instead and save your cell phone battery. Try to limit the use of wireless repeaters in the home. Replace wireless networks with wired alternatives to reduce the number of wireless radiation sources. This will probably improve network performance anyway as an added benefit. When it makes sense to do so, use wired devices in lieu of wireless counterparts.

*   *   *

For other situations at home and at work, treat wireless devices like you would any source of electricity. Continue to operate them as needed, but try to use common sense to minimize your exposure.

Preventing Neck and Back Problems

We spend an exorbitant amount of time using electronic devices, computers, and other electronic equipment within an office setting. The result is that our bodies are stagnant in unnatural positions for many hours. This kind of problem needs special attention, because it is something most of us deal with everyday due to work demands in an information-driven society. And it is a problem that is often ignored.

When many people use mobile electronic devices or laptop computers, their heads are tilted downward. And every inch the head is tilted in this way adds an enormous amount of pressure on the neck and spine [136]. Most people just don't think about the ramifications of this when they are texting, reading emails, or playing games.

In the short term, this irregular head posture can eventually lead to muscle strain, disc herniation, and pinched nerves. In the long term, it can actually change the natural curvature of the neck [137]. This type of damage can be cumulative, only manifesting itself years later in the form of chronic pain.

Furthermore, when people sit for long periods of time, overall body posture is out of alignment as well, affecting other parts of the spine and back. This is in addition to compounding health problems associated with inactivity in general. When we stay stationary in front of a computer or hunched over a mobile device, we spend less time walking, moving, and enjoying the outdoors.

Ultimately, this increases our risk of becoming immobile as we get older.

Consider the following recommendations when using electronic devices or computers for long periods of time. Much of this is common sense, but we often forget the basics.

When Sitting:

• Sit up straight and try to keep your back aligned with the chair. In general, the head should be level, forward facing, balanced, and aligned with the torso [138]. You can switch positions in the chair as long as you keep your back straight. Your lower legs should remain vertical with your feet flat on the floor. Avoid crossing your legs or sitting on them.

• Reduce neck and back strain by adjusting the computer monitor to your natural resting eye position. If the monitor doesn't adjust, there are desk stands that are adjustable.

• Adjust the font, resolution, and zoom (magnification) of onscreen text to allow for easy reading so you don't have to lead too far forward. The added benefit is that this will help prevent digital eye strain. If the text is still difficult to read, you may need to invest in corrective eye wear, not only for your eyes, but also to protect your neck and back in the long run.

• Consider acquiring a posture-friendly or ergonomic office chair designed for the amount of work you are doing. If you spend a significant amount of time in the seated position, it is probably worth spending some extra money on a quality chair. An alternative, and probably a less expensive option, is to acquire foot rests or lumbar support pads to improve your posture in an existing chair.

When Standing

• Keep your head up and try to maintain good alignment between your legs, shoulders, neck, and head [138]. Keep your shoulders back instead of hunched over to look at electronic devices or keyboards. Adjustable stand-up desks, work tables, or desk stands should help if you have to stay on your feet while using the equipment.

When Carrying Electronic Gear

• If carrying electronics in an arm bag or a case with a shoulder strap, don't overload it. If a bag or case is too heavy, it may be nearly impossible to stand or walk with proper alignment.

• If you are carrying a laptop in a backpack and you have to lean forward or to one side, it is too heavy. Consider lightening the load or, when all else fails, acquire a computer case with wheels.

• Consider spending extra money to purchase purses, bags, or backpacks that are specifically designed to minimize back strain, especially if carrying heavier electronic items.

When Using a Handheld Device

• Make sure you are not hunched over when using your smartphone or handheld device. Keep your feet flat on the ground, your shoulders back, and your ears directly over your shoulders to avoid constantly leaning forward [137]. You may need to train yourself to raise your smartphone closer to eye level to avoid looking down while it is in use. This should be easier to do with the availability of lighter materials in newer electronic devices. In fact, you should pay attention to the weight of the device you intend to purchase.

• Consider acquiring a hands-free headset to help maintain good posture while using your smart phone or having a conversation.

When Using any Electronic Device or Computer

• Take frequent short breaks. Whether you are using a computer or handheld device, you need to take multiple breaks each hour. Even while maintaining good posture, prolonged computer use will keep you in a relative state of physical inactivity, which has its own health dangers beyond the neck and back.

• During breaks, stretch, roll your shoulders, walk around, or get some fresh air. Doing so will give you more energy, reduce back and neck pain, and will even help avoid digital eye strain.

*   *   *

Following these basic guidelines should help with preventing neck and back pain at the very least. If you are not sure if you are addressing the problem correctly, there are some obvious signs that may indicate bad posture. For example, you may experience random discomfort at certain times of the day or week. It may go away after switching positions in a chair. It could also accompany a new job or a new chair. All of these are clues for self-diagnosis.

Since something like this could lead to a chronic condition later on, you can begin preventive measures now to resolve the problem as quickly as possible. However, it is important to note that if you are currently suffering from severe neck or back pain, only a doctor or a specialist can provide relief.

Putting it All Together

This chapter covered some of the more subtle ways modern technology affects our health.

Although much of the current research is inconclusive on the long-term health effects of electromagnetic radiation, we should take a precautionary approach while more studies are being conducted. This means limiting, as much as possible, any excessive exposure to all sources of radiation, even those with low power emissions.

We need to recognize that technology has changed the way we sit, stand, and walk. Since electronic devices and computers are now ubiquitous at work and around the home, we should pay more attention to our posture when interacting with these devices. Furthermore, since the same technology has the potential to make us inactive, we should compensate by increasing the number of breaks during long work hours and by staying physically active by any means necessary.

The following action steps can be taken right away to improve your health.

ACTION STEPS

1. Go <u>hands free</u> when using your <u>cell phone or other wireless device</u> by acquiring a <u>headset</u> or using the <u>speakerphone</u>. This will keep radiation exposure, especially near your head, at a minimum.

2. Respect <u>all EMF emitting devices and equipment</u> as <u>sources of electricity</u>. When you are done using them, put them away. Store and carry them <u>away from your body</u> unless you plan to use them in the near future.

3. Take <u>frequent breaks</u> while working long hours in front of a computer or using any portable electronic device in a seated position. Be sure to <u>stretch, walk, or go outside several times per hour</u>, if possible.

4. Become consciously <u>aware of your posture</u> when using mobile devices, sitting at a desk, or operating vehicles. Keep your <u>neck and back straight</u>. Acquire <u>ergonomic accessories</u> to make this task easier.

Chapter 9: Cosmetics and Skin Protection

Protecting Your Skin

When it comes to skin, there are a number of potential health threats that we are exposed to on a daily basis. We often overlook many of them. For example, personal care products, including cosmetics, contain chemical ingredients that can be absorbed by different layers of the skin and even end up in the bloodstream. The clothes that we wear every day contain chemicals that brush up against our skin. Also, too much ultraviolet radiation from the sun can increase our risk of skin cancers. There are even circumstances where skin products are contaminated by bacteria, which can lead to infection and illness. By being aware of these potential hazards, we can take precautionary measures to minimize exposure.

When it comes to skin exposure, the potential long-term **health problems** are as follows.

● Chronic inflammation can result from exposure to **toxic chemicals** and **bacteria** in cosmetics, personal care products, and in some cases, clothing. This can potentially increase the risk of chronic diseases such as **heart disease**, **diabetes**, **Alzheimer's disease**, **stroke**, **arthritis**, and certain types of **cancer**.

● Chronic inflammation, as a result of gradual buildup of trace chemicals in our bodies, and especially our skin, can increase our susceptibility to chronic diseases across-the-board, including several types of skin **cancer**.

● Excessive exposure to **ultraviolet radiation** from the sun or artificial sources can also increase our risk of **skin cancer** [7].

Chapter 9: Cosmetics and Skin Protection

*   *   *

So, we know there are many potentially harmful substances that we incidentally make contact with on a regular basis. And there are some that we purposely apply to our skin regularly. When we responsibly use such products or, in the case of ultraviolet radiation, engage in outdoor activities in a responsible manner, resultant exposure is unlikely to cause serious health problems. However, as with almost anything related to health, indiscriminate use (or excessive exposure) can increase our risk of chronic disease. Naturally, this risk is not uniform for all individuals. It can be increased or decreased based on genetic makeup. But, whether we possess good or bad genes, all of us should use common sense when it comes to our skin. After all, it is considered to be the largest organ of the body.

This chapter will cover personal care products, including cosmetics mainly. It will also address exposure to other hazards such as ultraviolet radiation from sun exposure.

When it comes to personal care products, cosmetics are an integral part of most people's lives, whether male or female. Cosmetics are meant to promote attractiveness or alter physical appearance in some way. They consist of a number of different products including perfumes, lipsticks, fingernail polishes, eye and facial makeup, cleansing shampoos, permanent waves, hair colors, deodorants, dental care products, tanning products, and many other substances. It may be surprising, but the companies that produce these products are solely responsible, in most respects, for their safety. Regulatory agencies are only responsible for certain types of chemical ingredients, such as artificial colors. It is for this reason that we must use these products responsibly and avoid overuse. We need to remember that what we use every day can have long-term consequences, even if the risks appear to be trivial in the short-term.

Luckily, it is not necessary to try to keep track of every chemical additive and hidden ingredient in personal care products. This would be near impossible anyway. Common sense measures to prevent overexposure to one type of chemical will also work well enough to minimize exposure to others. This is what we will focus on.

Signs of Skin Irritation

In the short term, there is often clear evidence of overexposure to chemicals and other substances. Some of the symptoms are listed in the following table (table 20) [139, 140]. These symptoms are caused by conditions that irritate, clog, or inflame the skin. Many common skin problems, such as dermatitis and hives, can be exacerbated by such skin conditions.

Redness	Pain	Wrinkles
Swelling	Stinging	Dry skin
Burning	Eye discharge	Scaling
Itchy skin	Blurred vision	Moles
Rashes	Small bumps	Sores

Table 20 – Signs of skin irritation. These symptoms may be the result of overexposure to chemicals and other substances.

Note that reactions to a chemical ingredient or other substance may not occur right away. As discussed previously, chemicals can build up over time in the body and, in the case of your skin, cause noticeable symptoms weeks or even months later. This can make self-diagnosis difficult and make the exact cause difficult to pinpoint. Furthermore, even if you stop using the offending product, or eliminate the source quickly, symptoms could continue to appear for a long time afterward. It depends on how fast your body can expel the foreign substance. It is important to understand that any skin condition that is allowed to continue unabated is, in itself, a form of chronic inflammation which we are trying to avoid.

Contamination of Cosmetics and Personal Care Products

Whether chemical or biological, contamination is always a problem in personal care products. On the chemical side, contamination can occur anytime during the manufacturing process or when the product is distributed and sold. We can also contaminate the products all on our own by mixing them with other substances intentionally or accidently.

But, chemicals are not the only contaminates of concern. Biological contaminates, such as bacteria, can also irritate the skin and cause infection. Even though cosmetics have preservatives to minimize the bacteria present, new bacteria can be introduced from the air and from dirty hands, applicators, and surfaces. The older the cosmetic, the less effective the preservatives are.

To minimize exposure to both types of contaminates, precautionary measures need to be employed [141, 142]. Of course, most of this can be considered common sense, but it is important to reiterate how important these measures are in preventing chronic diseases and other long-term health problems.

● **Throw old cosmetic products away** – Note that cosmetics are not required by law to have expiration dates, so in some cases, you'll have to keep track of that yourself. In this case, it pays to buy what you need and only when you need it. The estimated shelf life of common makeup products is shown in table 21.

Product Type	Estimated Shelf-life
Mascara	2 to 3 months
Eyeliner	4 to 6 months
Eye creams or face creams	4 to 6 months
Lipsticks and lip liners	1 to 2 years
Eye shadow	Up to 3 years
Blush	Up to 3 years
Face powder, powdered products	Up to 3 years

Table 21 – Estimated shelf life of common cosmetic products. Note that cosmetics are not required by law to have expiration dates, so in some cases, you'll have to keep track of that yourself.

• **Throw potentially contaminated products away** – If the product exhibits an unexpected change in smell, color, or texture, it may be safer to throw that product away. The sudden change could indicate a chemical reaction or the presence of bacteria due to nonfunctioning preservatives. The aspect of color, however, does not apply to certain makeup creams or liquids that darken naturally when exposed to air.

• **Avoid application near breaks in the skin** – If you have a cut or scrape near the area of application, it is best to avoid cosmetics or skin care products at that location. Breaks in the skin are a direct route to the bloodstream and can make irritation worse. This also applies to open skin conditions such as active eczema. Unless applying a cream that specifically treats eczema, avoid applying any sort of skin care or cosmetic product to the area.

• **Wash your hands before and after application** – Clean your hands before you handle or apply makeup or other skin care products. Wash afterwards so that you do not continue distributing the chemical.

• **Keep the area sanitized and the applicators clean** – Clean and sanitize bathroom countertops before items are placed on them. Wash makeup brushes regularly with soap and water. You can also use sanitizing cleaners for those products.

• **Do not mistakenly contaminate makeup** – You need to keep the product as pure as possible. One of the easier ways to prevent contamination is not to share makeup with others. Note that department store cosmetic counters were found to be even more likely to be contaminated than cosmetics in the home, according to tests. So, when in stores, insist only on the use of disposable single-use applicators.

As for self-contamination, if you have an eye infection, stay away from eye makeup and throw away any makeup that was used when you discovered it. If you have a cold sore on your lip, cut off and dispose of the top layer of lip balms after you apply it. Don't directly touch any makeup in its original container. Instead, you should pour it out into the palm of your hand or scoop a little out with a clean disposable applicator such as a sponge or spoon, and then make sure the applicator is clean before reintroducing it to the container. Obviously, don't put your fingers into the container either.

• **Don't mix products or add water** – Unless indicated in the instructions, do not mix chemicals. Also, do not add water to liquid cosmetics. The water may contain bacteria that could contaminate the product. Water can also affect the chemical makeup of the cosmetic and cause irritation. Similarly, don't add moisture such as saliva to eye cosmetics.

• **Store products safely** – Don't expose containers to extreme temperature. In particular, don't store products in temperatures above 85 degrees Fahrenheit. Keep containers clean. Don't leave brushes, applicators, or eyelash wands on the bathroom countertop where they can be contaminated by moisture from the sink.

Reducing Chemical Exposure

To prevent chronic inflammation, we need to minimize exposure to chemicals that touch our skin throughout the day.

There are thousands of chemicals present in cosmetics and skin care products. Many are added to improve coloring, texture, and smell, as well as function as preservatives. With new products coming out all the time, it is almost impossible to keep track of every new chemical added. Take, for example, the fact that hair dyes in general have over five thousand different chemicals in them [143]. No one will have time to do sufficient research on all those chemicals. Also, industry is largely responsible for self-regulating the safety of these products. Except for color additives, cosmetics don't go through an approval process before they are released to market. So, obviously, we will not be able to avoid all exposure. However, we are responsible for how much exposure we subject ourselves to.

To avoid overexposure of natural or synthetic chemicals, the following common sense guidelines apply.

• **Don't use more than you need** – Whether you are using products such as toothpaste, deodorant, makeup, or any other personal care product, be a minimalist. Use exactly what is necessary and no more. The instructions on the packaging should help determine what amount of product to use. If you have ignored these instructions in the past, just keep in mind that some personal care products, such as antiperspirants, are classified as over-the-counter drugs! And using too much of any drug can have unintended side effects.

• **Don't use these products too often** – Only use products as often as needed and no more than recommended by the manufacturer. You need to keep your body clean and free of added chemicals whenever possible. For example, to minimize unnecessary exposure, put on cosmetic makeup just before you expect to go out. And, avoid wearing makeup for extended periods of time.

● **Use only as directed** – Don't use any cosmetic or personal care product for anything other than what it was designed for. For example, don't get creative and use a lip liner as an eye liner. And always read the instructions to ensure you are using it properly.

● **Use only reputable company products** – Because cosmetic and personal care products are not strictly regulated, you should not necessarily trust everything you buy. You are essentially relying on the manufacturer's reputation and good will for safety. A well-established and reputable company will have a proven track record that includes processing customer complaints in a professional and timely manner. Otherwise, that company would not have survived as long as it did. If you are not sure about a product, or if the company is relatively new, consider verifying that color additives and other ingredients on the label are approved for safety. A list of approved color additives can be found on the Food and Drug Administration website [144]. Note that if the cosmetic does not have an ingredients label at all, it is illegal and misbranded. Avoid these unlabeled products and the parent company entirely.

● **Minimize time of exposure** – When you are done using makeup or any other removable cosmetic product, remove it as soon as you can. Over time, some of the product will evaporate, and some will be absorbed by the skin. You want to minimize the amount that is absorbed, since too much may end up in deeper layers of the skin and perhaps the bloodstream.

● **Consider washing up and bathing before bed** – Chemicals from personal care products and clothing can be transferred to the skin and linger all night long. Get in the habit of washing your hands and face before bed at the very least. You may even consider bathing or showering to remove surface chemicals on the rest of your body. Regardless of your evening cleaning ritual, do not wear makeup to bed. Use makeup remover or wash it off beforehand.

● **Look for less toxic ingredients and use homemade alternatives** – Try to use less toxic products. Less toxic products typically have fewer ingredients, including some with more natural properties, but note that this is not always the case. Some synthetic ingredients, especially those that have been around a long time, have been demonstrated to be relatively safe. However, when the opportunity presents itself and it is safe to do so, try to use homemade alternatives in place of commercial products. For example, you may try jojoba oil as a makeup remover or baking soda as a mouthwash [145].

When in doubt about a product with a large and confusing chemical ingredients list, remember to use as little of the product as necessary. From the standpoint of health, the numerous chemicals contained within are likely to cause some form of skin irritation, especially if overused.

• **Stop using products that irritate the skin** – If you exhibit signs of skin irritation, stop using the product that is most likely causing it. Of course, this may not be obvious at first. It could be months later before a certain cosmetic or personal care product builds up in the system and causes noticeable symptoms. So, you may have to use some trial and error. However, if the condition worsens or persists, it may be prudent to talk to your healthcare provider. No doubt, repeated exposure to the same toxic ingredients will worsen whatever condition you are experiencing.

*　　*　　*

Remember the safest route when using cosmetics and any other personal care product is to follow the manufacturer's instructions and limit, through moderation, overall exposure as much as you can.

Chemicals in Clothing

We wear clothing every day. Yet, we give little thought about the fact that this material is touching our bodies twenty-four hours a day. Clothing is produced with chemicals. Through chemical treatments, they are flame-retardant, made to look like a certain color, are wrinkle-free and static-free, and are often scented before placement on the shelves. They are manufactured in machines that are cleaned with potent chemicals and these may end up in the final product before distributed in stores. Some of the chemicals, such as formaldehyde, are very toxic and are known to be carcinogenic [146]. And yet still, many of these same clothes are produced overseas, where manufacturers are under less scrutiny than in the United States and are under no obligation to divulge what chemicals are being used in the manufacturing process.

Regardless of where clothes are manufactured, it is advisable that **whenever you purchase new clothes**, that you **wash them at least once**, and **preferably multiple times before wearing them**. Over time, such contaminates dissipate of course, but while you are wearing the clothing, you are being exposed to substances that may be harmful to long-term health. Thorough washing is necessary to flush out the majority of chemicals and other contaminates from the clothing that you plan to wear regularly.

In reference to washing out chemicals, you should also strive to use more natural detergents, or even homemade detergents, whenever you can. Even though water dilutes whatever chemicals are in the cleaning solution, more natural ingredients are preferable to synthetic counterparts for the same reason we want to avoid contact with similar chemicals in clothing. Furthermore, when you do wash clothes, follow the instructions closely, and use only the minimum amount of a cleaning solution as necessary. This is how we minimize exposure the easy way. Remember that this material is touching our skin throughout the day.

If you are having a reaction, consider the fact that clothing could be the culprit, especially if it was just purchased from the store.

Reducing Ultraviolet Radiation Exposure

Everyone knows that sunlight enables our bodies to produce vitamin D, which is critical to health. Unfortunately, too much of a good thing has its drawbacks, even when it applies to something completely natural. Unnecessary sun exposure can cause long-term skin damage, which could lead to skin cancer. In fact, over 3 million cases of skin cancer per year are attributed to ultraviolet rays from the sun [147]. This statistic suggests that we need to limit exposure greatly. And it is important to remember that we can always get enough vitamin D from eating nutrient-dense foods or foods fortified with vitamin D. Don't try to spend more time in the sun for the sake of health.

To minimize sun exposure, consider the following recommendations [148, 149].

• **Select the right sunscreen** – Broad-spectrum commercial sunscreens with SPF 30 or better will block 97% of all ultraviolet rays. Higher SPF (sun protection factor) levels only result in marginal increases in protection. For example, SPF 50 would only block 98% of all ultraviolet rays, so going higher does not necessary translate to proportionately better protection. SPF 30 is the recommended level for outdoor activities. If you are expecting to go into the water, look for water-resistant varieties. Also note that a lotion will likely provide better uniform coverage than a spray.

Be careful when experimenting with homemade sunscreens and other remedies. Although they may be cheaper and may appear to be less toxic, they have not been tested for effectiveness and may expose you to increased risk.

• **Apply sunscreen as often as you need it** – Sunscreen should be reapplied **at least every two hours during outdoor activities**. You'll need to apply more if you are sweating or getting in and out of the water. It is also recommended that you do the first application **fifteen minutes before starting outdoor activities**. Note that if you are around water, snow, and sand, you are at a greater risk of sunburn due to the combined reflections of the sun's rays.

• **Avoid excessive exposure** – Stay indoors or stay under shade between the hours of ten and four during the day. This is when ultraviolet rays are strongest. Note that sunburns are a clear sign of damage to the skin. Also, note that radiation can go through clouds and fog, so don't assume protection during cloudy days.

• **Use protective clothing** – Cover up exposed parts of the body with clothing, a hat, and sunglasses, especially on hot sunny days. To protect your eyes, be sure the sunglasses are broad spectrum, which protects from several types of ultraviolet rays (UVA and UVB).

• **Avoid artificial sources of ultraviolet radiation** – Avoid tanning booths, for they can concentrate ultraviolet radiation at an intensity that is much greater than that of the sun. As a result, they increase the likelihood of developing sunburn.

*   *   *

Not all people will be affected by ultraviolet radiation in the same way. For example, people with a family history of skin cancer or those who have pale skin need to be very careful when engaging in activities outdoors. Still, regardless of your history or skin type, you can prevent skin damage and dramatically decrease your risk of skin cancer by taking proper precautions and limiting sun exposure.

Tattoos and Long-Term Health

Tattoos seem to be very popular as of late. But, the effect on long-term health is a bit of a mystery to many. It should be noted that tattoos have not been approved by the Food and Drug Administration and this is the first warning flag. The second is the fact that many of the pigments used in tattoo inks are suitable for industrial-grade applications such as printing, or painting of automobiles [150]. This fact alone should give you pause on exposing yourself to such chemicals over so many years.

Of course, studies are being conducted to evaluate short and long-term safety issues, including the chemical composition of the inks, as well as how the body reacts to them under the skin.

The potential health-related ramifications of tattoos include:

• Allergic reaction, or irritation, to the ink pigments (e.g. rashes, itching, or swelling) that can last months or even years [151]

• Breakdown of tattoo pigments into toxic components that may disperse throughout the body

• Rejection of the ink as a foreign substance, leading to chronic inflammation

• Risk of infection and diseases such as hepatitis and HIV from dirty needles

• Permanent scarring around tattoos

*   *   *

Unless you surgically remove them, you will likely have your tattoos for your entire life. The best advice is to largely avoid them, especially the permanent ones, until more conclusive studies are conducted to determine that they are medically safe for the long-term.

Hand Sanitizers and Antibacterial Soaps

For sanitary reasons, we are told to wash our hands often. We are also told that hand sanitizers and antibacterial soaps will make our hands cleaner and free from bacteria. Unfortunately, constant use of such products can also adversely affect our health.

Hand sanitizers and antibacterial soaps have chemical ingredients, and, like other personal care products, can result in the same hidden dangers. Not only that, they can make existing skin conditions such as eczema and dermatitis worse with repeated use. It is important to note these risks because of the prevalence of these products and how they are marketed. The Food and Drug Administration even warns against excessive use and is considering a ban on certain chemicals [152].

There are numerous hand sanitizers and antibacterial soaps out there and they all offer protection against germs. However, the effectiveness is being questioned and many products are unproven against more resistant germs such as MRSA. Even the claim about protection against 99.9% of germs should be considered suspicious and most likely exaggerated [153]. The truth is that regular soap and water work just fine for the same purpose, by removing germs of all types from the surface of skin.

As a rule, you should always use regular soap and water to disinfect and only use hand sanitizers and antibacterial soaps as a last resort. So, exposure to the chemicals contained in these products is largely unnecessary. When you do wash your hands with regular soap, be sure to rub your hands together vigorously to dislodge bacteria-containing dirt and particles.

If you do use chemicals to disinfect your hands or bathe, you may want to avoid known irritants such as triclosan in liquid soaps and hand sanitizers, and triclocarban in bar soaps. Both should be clearly identified on the product label. For these popular chemicals, long-term health effects have not been fully evaluated and studies are ongoing. Keep in mind that the only reason you should use such products to protect from germs is because you have no other option.

By simply restricting the use of hand sanitizers and antibacterial products, you are minimizing your exposure to potentially harmful substances while still protecting yourself from the most harmful germs.

Putting it All Together

It is probably a good idea to treat cosmetic and personal care products like food. In a sense, both can cause inflammation if an individual is overexposed to added ingredients or harmful contaminates. Remember the skin is a major organ after all. It is common sense to use such products sparingly.

Additionally, we need to realize that clothing can contain harmful chemicals. As a result, such chemicals can touch our skin for long periods of time. To reduce exposure, clothing should be washed thoroughly before wearing them, especially when they are newly manufactured.

Of course, when it comes to skin irritation and long-term health, chemicals aren't the only concern. We also need to be aware of the total time we spend in the sun. We should not intentionally increase this time for nutritional purposes. Instead, we should get the nutrients we need from a healthy diet. When we go outside, especially for extended activities, we need to minimize exposure to ultraviolet radiation as much as possible.

The following action steps can be taken right away to improve your health.

ACTION STEPS

1. Limit use of cosmetics and personal care products to a minimum. Do not use more than you need. Always follow the instructions on the product label and use only as directed.

2. Wash new clothes at least once, preferably multiple times, before you wear them.

3. Limit time in the sun and be sure to use an effective sunscreen. Broad spectrum sunscreens should be SPF 30 or better for outdoor activities. Consider using protective clothing to further reduce risk.

4. Avoid using hand sanitizers and antibacterial soaps, which contain potentially harmful chemicals. Use regular soap and water to wash your hands and bathe. Only use personal sanitizing products as a last resort to kill germs.

Conclusion

In this book, we have addressed methods to prevent chronic diseases and debilitating conditions using practical approaches along with a dose of common sense. You do have the power to change your state of health and your long-term fate. It should now be clear how your actions in the present can have a profound effect on your future. To live a long and productive life, we all need to focus on risk factors that really matter. This is easier to accomplish with a comprehensive system, one that is seamlessly integrated into our lifestyles.

Being proactive also means being both consistent and persistent. The tools to make this happen are right in front of us. We do not have to rely solely on healthcare professionals or the medical system as a whole to do the work for us. Even if we did, the results would not be good enough to ward off long-term chronic health problems. The truth is: <u>**we are responsible for ourselves**</u>. It is our responsibility to avoid the vicious circle of chronic disease and disability. Ignoring the threats that surround us in a modern world may get some sympathy later on, but it will lead to few solutions. Additionally, we must take action as soon as possible. Time is of the essence.

At this point, you have already increased your knowledge and therefore your odds of success when it comes to long-term health. Hopefully, this book has strengthened, if not generated, a **mindset** to do what is necessary to live longer and healthier. Before closing, however, let's discuss a few more important recommendations.

- **Focus on what is really important** – As human beings, we have a tendency to overcomplicate our lives. When it comes to the things we want in life, it is often said that most of the results we get come from just a fraction of the input we produce. When it comes to managing chronic disease, the same can be said about reducing risk.

It is very tempting to try some exotic health regimen as a convenient short-term approach to improve your vitality and long-term health. However, if at the same time, you are carrying around an excessive amount of weight, for example, the new health regimen will probably not make much difference in preventing heart disease or diabetes down-the-road. You need to focus on the things that really matter. With regard to weight gain, obesity is such a strong indicator of chronic disease that you should probably put all of your physical, mental, emotional, and spiritual energy into getting your weight under control first. Once you have taken care of that, you can try adding secondary remedies or lifestyle changes that have a lower probability of working. Be sure to prioritize.

The glaringly obvious problems are the ones that should be tackled first. The primary risk factors listed in the introduction have to be minimized at all costs.

- **Address potential problems early** – For reasons already discussed throughout the book, we need to take action to minimize the risk of chronic diseases and other conditions as early as possible in our lives. Although there is plenty of research being done to understand the triggers of chronic disease, we still do not fully know how stressors encountered today affect our lives decades into the future. Regardless of when you start, even if you are already suffering from one or more chronic conditions, now is not the time to delay or otherwise terminate action you started. It is never too late to improve health, for the impact of current chronic conditions can still be lessened through immediate lifestyle changes. However, the research of epigenetics is uncovering how our lifestyle and our environment influence the behavior of our genes, and by extension, the resiliency of our bodies over the course of our lives. The implication of this is that strengthening our bodies and changing persistent habits over the long term will have more potential benefit if started earlier rather than attempted at the last minute.

- **Remember that science is work-in-progress** – There is no doubt we will continue to get barraged with new information about health every day. It can be overwhelming if we don't already have a plan or some way of extracting what is relevant. When dealing with this reality, the important thing to remember is that science is work-in-progress. To explain, it takes time for new studies to be applied and then verified by the scientific community. Then, all studies need follow-up with other studies to uncover the validity of a particular health claim. You cannot take the health claim from one study at face value. To make matters worse, single health studies are often sensationalized by the media and, as a result, misunderstood. Worse yet, some studies only apply to animals. Just because the latest health experiment worked on a lab animal does not mean it will come close to working in the human body. It only gives a starting point for more investigation, and that type of investigation could take years. Putting full faith in early results is a waste of time, money, and may even jeopardize your health if you jump onboard too early. Most of the information in this book, therefore, is based on time-tested, rigorously-studied concepts and recommendations.

The risk factors presented early in this book, for instance, are clear threats to health because they are based on numerous studies which have achieved a consensus in the scientific community over a long period of time. We can be confident that some kind of connection exists between chronic diseases and these risk factors for a vast majority of the population. Keep this in mind when you go out and do your own research on the Internet.

Furthermore, watch out for anecdotal evidence based on personal observations of your friends, neighbors, and other media, including Internet sources. Even if a recommendation has merit, there may be other variables at play besides the new supplement, new diet, or health regimen they are currently advocating. And don't forget about the placebo effect. Belief in something can be so strong that a particular remedy can appear to have a health benefit when there actually isn't one.

● **Be happy, enjoy life, and stay positive** – The mental aspect of health, especially long-term health, is a bit of a wild card. Although difficult to measure and tough to teach, it still appears to have a major effect on overall health. It is no surprise that we all need to smile more, laugh more, be happier, and think positive. Furthermore, you will find that this state of mind is contagious. The result to you and others around you is lower stress, which in itself may be the greatest secret to health and longevity. When centenarians (people who live past one hundred years of age) are asked what their secret to long life is, they often attribute their longevity to being happy, enjoying life, and feeling younger [154].

This confirms what many of us probably suspected already. The body and mind work together, so it is not a stretch to conclude that a negative mindset could result in our bodies failing us in the form of chronic disease. It will certainly, at the very least, prevent you from taking care of yourself properly. While being optimistic and happy keeps these centenarians going, some of their longevity is obviously the result of good genes. But, we have already discussed how we can somewhat compensate for this, so don't let bad genes discourage you.

Earlier in this book, we also discussed the danger of stress over the long term. The obvious way to counter stress is to change one's state of mind or do something productive that keeps the mind off the stress.

This may be a good time to mention that utilizing complementary and alternative medicine (CAM) techniques is a great way to augment any steps that you take to ensure that the mind stays healthy. At chronic disease treatment centers around the country, such methods are employed, in addition to traditional medicine, to help patients heal or rehabilitate. Techniques such as yoga, meditation, tai chi, aromatherapy, acupuncture, hydrotherapy, and others can help relieve symptoms of disease, stimulate the healing process, help achieve greater levels of relaxation, and improve mood [155]. It doesn't matter how you achieve a positive mental state, as long as it is done in a healthy manner. In fact, you should try every trick in the book to maintain a healthy outlook on life. That is why it is important not to discount such alternative methods. They can potentially make a difference.

*   *   *

Conclusion

Hopefully, you have found the information in this book useful. It has been researched and consolidated to be relevant and easy to understand. Now, it is important that you integrate it into your self-care system to achieve better health and a longer life. It is worth noting that maintaining a relationship with your physician or healthcare provider is equally important and is imperative. Without such a relationship, a physician or healthcare provider cannot fully support you in your quest to stay proactive and address health concerns early. It is just another tool you have available to you, and you should use it.

Finally, don't just put this book down and go on with life as usual. Make it a tool for you and your family to invest in health in a way that is fun, simple, and convenient. If you take some steps now, the odds will likely be stacked in your favor later when you need it most.

Good luck and here's hoping we all get to be healthy and happy centenarians.

Bibliography

[1]   Centers for Disease Control and Prevention, "Deaths and Mortality,"
        6 February 2015. [Online]. Available:
        http://www.cdc.gov/nchs/fastats/deaths.htm.

[2]   Centers for Disease Control and Prevention, "Prevalence and Most
        Common Causes of Disability Among Adults, United States, 2005," 1
        May 2009. [Online]. Available:
        http://www.cdc.gov/mmwr/preview/mmwrhtml/mm5816a2.htm.

[3]   World Health Organization, "Diet, Nutrition, and the Prevention of
        Chronic Diseases Report of the Joint WHO/FAO Expert Consultation,"
        2015. [Online]. Available:
        http://www.who.int/dietphysicalactivity/publications/trs916/summ
        ary/en/.

[4]   Public Health Agency of Canada, "Arthritis Risk Factors," 20 August
        2010. [Online]. Available: http://www.phac-aspc.gc.ca/cd-
        mc/arthritis-arthrite/risk-risque-eng.php.

[5]   Australian Institute if Health and Welfare, "Risk Factors Contributing
        to Chronic Disease," Australian Institute if Health and Welfare,
        Canberra, Australia, 2012.

[6]   Centers for Disease Control and Prevention, "Obesity Halting the
        Epidemic by Making Health Easier," Centers for Disease Control and
        Prevention, Atlanta, GA, 2011.

[7]   American Academy of Dermatology, "Skin Cancer: Who Gets and
        Causes," 2015. [Online]. Available:
        https://www.aad.org/dermatology-a-to-z/diseases-and-
        treatments/q---t/skin-cancer/who-gets-causes. [Accessed 1 January

2015].

[8]   Centers for Disease Control and Prevention, "Sleep and Chronic
        Disease," 1 July 2013. [Online]. Available:
        http://www.cdc.gov/sleep/about_sleep/chronic_disease.htm.

[9]   C. J. Schoessow, "Family and Consumer Services, Type 2 Diabetes
        Basics," 9 December 2014. [Online]. Available:
        http://fcs.tamu.edu/health/type_2_diabetes/type_2_diabetes_basic
        s.php.

[10]   G. Reynolds, "How Exercise Changes our DNA," 17 December 2014.
        [Online]. Available: http://well.blogs.nytimes.com/2014/12/17/how-
        exercise-changes-our-dna/.

[11]   U.S. Department of Agriculture, U.S. Department of Health and
        Human Services, "Dietary Guidelines for Americans 2010 7th
        Edition," U.S. Government Printing Office, Washington, DC, 2010.

[12]   J. Di Noia, "Defining Powerhouse Fruits and Vegetables: A Nutrient
        Density Approach," 5 June 2014. [Online]. Available:
        http://www.cdc.gov/pcd/issues/2014/13_0390.htm.

[13]   U.S. Department of Health and Human Services, "Your Guide to
        Lowering Blood Pressure," 2003. [Online]. Available:
        http://www.nhlbi.nih.gov/files/docs/public/heart/hbp_low.pdf.
        [Accessed 1 January 2015].

[14]   U.S. Department of Health and Human Services, "Your Guide to
        Lowering Your Cholesterol with TLC," 2005. [Online]. Available:
        http://www.nhlbi.nih.gov/files/docs/public/heart/chol_tlc.pdf.
        [Accessed 1 January 2015].

[15]   University of Wisconsin Hospitals and Clinics Authority,
        "Mediterranean Diet – Food Guide," November 2009. [Online].
        Available: http://www.uhs.wisc.edu/health-topics/healthy-

lifestyle/documents/Mediterranean.pdf. [Accessed 1 June 2015].

[16] Harvard University School of Public Health, "Healthy Eating Plate and Healthy Eating Pyramid," 2011. [Online]. Available: http://www.hsph.harvard.edu/nutritionsource/healthy-eating-plate/.

[17] Centers for Disease Control and Prevention, "Balancing Calories," 15 January 2014. [Online]. Available: http://www.cdc.gov/healthyweight/calories/.

[18] C. Gann and S. Albin, "For Calories, It's All About Quality Over Quantity, Harvard Study Says," 26 June 2012. [Online]. Available: http://abcnews.go.com/Health/calorie-calorie-harvard-study-compares-popular-weight-loss/story?id=16654506.

[19] U.S. News and World Report, "Best Diets 2015," 2015. [Online]. Available: http://health.usnews.com/best-diet.

[20] C. Cooper, "Drink Water to Cut Obesity, Health Experts Say," 25 June 2014. [Online]. Available: http://www.independent.co.uk/life-style/health-and-families/health-news/drink-water-to-cut-obesity-health-experts-say-9562887.html.

[21] Health.com, "The 10 Most Filling Foods for Weight Loss," 26 February 2014. [Online]. Available: http://time.com/9973/the-10-most-filling-foods-for-weight-loss/. [Accessed 2015].

[22] D. Stipp, "How Intermittent Fasting Might Help You Live a Longer and Healthier Life," 18 December 2012. [Online]. Available: http://www.scientificamerican.com/article/how-intermittent-fasting-might-help-you-live-longer-healthier-life. [Accessed 2015].

[23] L. Allen, B. de Benoist, O. Dary and R. Hurrell, "Guidelines on Food Fortification with Micronutrients," World Health Organization and Food and Agriculture Organization of the United Nations, Geneva,

Switzerland, 2006.

[24] CBC News, "Antioxidant Overload Can Be Hazardous," CBC News, 28 August 2013. [Online]. Available: http://www.cbc.ca/news/health/antioxidant-supplement-overload-can-be-hazardous-1.1412993.

[25] University of Colorado Denver, "Dietary Supplements Increase Cancer Risk," 15 May 2012. [Online]. Available: http://www.ucdenver.edu/about/newsroom/newsreleases/Pages/di etary-supplements-increase-cancer-risk.aspx.

[26] U.S. Food and Drug Administration, "Questions and Answers on Dietary Supplements," 28 April 2015. [Online]. Available: http://www.fda.gov/food/dietarysupplements/qadietarysupplement s/default.htm.

[27] World Health Organization and Food and Agriculture Organization of the United Nations, "Vitamins and Mineral Requirements in Human Nutrition 2nd Edition," World Health Organization and Food and Agriculture Organization of the United Nations, Geneva, Switzerland, 1998.

[28] U.S. Department of Agriculture, Agricultural Research Service, "USDA National Nutrient Database for Standard Reference, Release 27," 2 September 2014. [Online]. Available: http://www.ars.usda.gov/Services/docs.htm?docid=8964.

[29] University of Maryland Medical Center, "Complimentary and Alternative Medicine Guide," 31 July 2013. [Online]. Available: http://umm.edu/health/medical/altmed.

[30] U.S. National Library of Medicine, "Herbs and Supplements," 2015. [Online]. Available: http://www.nlm.nih.gov/medlineplus/druginfo/herb_All.html.

[Accessed 12 May 2015].

[31]   Therapeutic Research Faculty, "Natural Medicines Comprehensive
        Database," 2015. [Online]. Available:
        http://naturaldatabase.therapeuticresearch.com/Content.aspx?cs=&
        s=ND&page=edprinciples&xsl=generic. [Accessed 12 May 2015].

[32]   L. Landro, "The New Science Behind America's Deadliest Diseases,"
        16 July 2012. [Online]. Available:
        http://www.wsj.com/articles/SB10001424052702303612804577531
        092453590070. [Accessed 2015].

[33]   U.S. Food and Drug Administration, "Proposed Changes to the
        Nutrition Facts Label," 1 August 2014. [Online]. Available:
        http://www.fda.gov/Food/GuidanceRegulation/GuidanceDocuments
        RegulatoryInformation/LabelingNutrition/ucm385663.htm.

[34]   Clemson Cooperative Extension, "Reading the New Food Labels,"
        2015. [Online]. Available:
        http://www.clemson.edu/extension/hgic/food/nutrition/nutrition/di
        etary_guide/hgic4056.html.

[35]   C. Rivette, "Food Labels 101: Understanding the Nutrition Facts
        Panel," 28 April 2013. [Online]. Available:
        http://msue.anr.msu.edu/news/food_labels_101_understanding_th
        e_nutrition_facts_panel.

[36]   A. L. Ford and W. J. Dahl, "Functional Foods, FSHN12-17," November
        2012. [Online]. Available: http://edis.ifas.ufl.edu/fs210.

[37]   U.S. Department of Agriculture, Agriculture Research Service,
        "National Organic Program," 17 October 2012. [Online]. Available:
        http://www.ams.usda.gov/AMSv1.0/ams.fetchTemplateData.do?te
        mplate=TemplateC&navID=NationalOrganicProgram&leftNav=Natio
        nalOrganicProgram&page=NOPConsumers&description=Consumers

&acct=nopgeninfo.

[38]   Illinois Department of Agriculture, "Eggs: A Consumer Guide," 2001. [Online]. Available: http://www.agr.state.il.us/programs/consumer/egg/eggconsguide.html.

[39]   P. D. Tom and P. G. Olin, "Farmed or Wild? Both Types of Salmon Taste Good and are Good for You," June 2010. [Online]. Available: http://seafood.oregonstate.edu/.pdf%20Links/Farmed%20or%20Wild%20-%20Both%20Types%20of%20Salmon%20taste%20Good%20and%20Are%20Good%20For%20You.pdf.

[40]   U.S. Food and Drug Administration, "FDA Defines Gluten-Free on Food Labeling," 2 August 2013. [Online]. Available: http://www.fda.gov/NewsEvents/Newsroom/PressAnnouncements/ucm363474.htm.

[41]   M. Kimball , "Whole Grain or Whole Wheat Labels Can be Misleading," 26 February 2013. [Online]. Available: http://www.nola.com/health/index.ssf/2013/02/when_whole_grain_isnt.html.

[42]   Whole Grains Council, "Whole Grain Stamp," 2013. [Online]. Available: http://wholegrainscouncil.org. [Accessed 1 January 2013].

[43]   Clemson Cooperative Extension, "Nutrient Claims on Food Labels," 2015. [Online]. Available: http://www.clemson.edu/extension/hgic/food/nutrition/nutrition/dietary_guide/hgic4061.html.

[44]   U.S. Food and Drug Administration, "Guidance for Industry, A Food Labeling Guide," January 2013. [Online]. Available: http://www.fda.gov/Food/GuidanceRegulation/GuidanceDocuments

RegulatoryInformation/LabelingNutrition/ucm2006828.htm.

[45]   State Government of Victoria, "Food Processing and Nutrition,"
         September 2012. [Online]. Available:
         http://www.betterhealth.vic.gov.au/bhcv2/bhcarticles.nsf/pages/Fo
         od_processing_and_nutrition?open.

[46]   D. M. Barrett, "Maximizing the Nutritional Value of Fruits and
         Vegetables," *Food Technology* , pp. 61(4):40-44, 2007.

[47]   S. Bastin, "Chemical Cuisine, Commonly Used Food Additives from A-
         Z," January 2000. [Online]. Available:
         http://www2.ca.uky.edu/hes/fcs/factshts/FN-SSB.144.PDF.

[48]   International Food Information Council Foundation and U.S. Food
         and Drug Administration, "Food Ingredients and Colors," April 2010.
         [Online]. Available:
         http://www.foodinsight.org/Food_Ingredients_Colors.

[49]   W. D. Burgess and A. C. Mason, "What are All Those Chemicals in My
         Food?," September 1992. [Online]. Available:
         https://www.extension.purdue.edu/extmedia/HE/HE-625.html.

[50]   U.S. Food and Drug Administration, "GRAS Substances Database," 18
         March 2015. [Online]. Available:
         http://www.fda.gov/Food/IngredientsPackagingLabeling/GRAS/SCO
         GS/default.htm.

[51]   S. Polizzi, "Food Allergies and Intolerances," June 2013. [Online].
         Available:
         http://extension.oregonstate.edu/coos/sites/default/files/Fcd/docu
         ments/food_allergies.pdf.

[52]   Food Allergy Research and Education, "About Food Allergies," 2015.
         [Online]. Available: http://www.foodallergy.org/.

[53] University of Kentucky College of Agriculture, "Chemical Cuisine Commonly Used Food Additives from A-Z," January 2000. [Online]. Available: http://www2.ca.uky.edu/hes/fcs/factshts/FN-SSB.144.PDF. [Accessed 2015].

[54] University of Arizona, College of Agriculture and Life Sciences, "Food Additives - Are They Safe?," 2006. [Online]. Available: http://ag.arizona.edu/pubs/health/foodsafety/az1082.html.

[55] Oregon State University, "Older Adults and Pesticides," December 2011. [Online]. Available: http://npic.orst.edu/factsheets/olderadults.html.

[56] CBS News, "Lawn Chemicals Can Stay in the Body for Years, Even Decades," 25 July 2014. [Online]. Available: http://www.cbsnews.com/news/lawn-chemicals-can-stay-in-human-body-for-years-even-decades/.

[57] Environmental Working Group, "EWG's 2015 Shopper's Guide to Pesticides in Produce," 2015. [Online]. Available: http://www.ewg.org/foodnews/summary.php.

[58] U.S. Food and Drug Administration, "What You Need to Know About Mercury in Fish and Shellfish," 10 June 2014. [Online]. Available: http://www.fda.gov/Food/FoodborneIllnessContaminants/Metals/ucm351781.htm.

[59] U.S. Food and Drug Administration, "Questions and Answers: Arsenic in Rice and Rice Products," 4 August 2014. [Online]. Available: http://www.fda.gov/Food/FoodborneIllnessContaminants/Metals/ucm319948.htm.

[60] J. Schilling and D. Lee, "California Food Guide, Enivornmental Contaminants in Food," 10 January 2006. [Online]. Available: http://www.dhcs.ca.gov/formsandpubs/publications/CaliforniaFood

Guide/26EnvironmentalContaminants.pdf.

[61]   University of Kentucky College of Agriculture, "Preserving Nutrients in Food," February 2000. [Online]. Available: http://www2.ca.uky.edu/HES/fcs/factshts/FN-SSB.006.PDF. [Accessed 2015].

[62]   The New York Times, "Preserving the Nutrients of Food with Proper Care," 7 July 1982. [Online]. Available: http://www.nytimes.com/1982/07/07/garden/preserving-the-nutrients-of-food-with-proper-care.html. [Accessed 1 January 2015].

[63]   J. Nelson, "Is Juicing Healthier Than Eating Whole Fruits or Vegetables?," 30 January 2014. [Online]. Available: http://www.mayoclinic.org/healthy-living/nutrition-and-healthy-eating/expert-answers/juicing/faq-20058020. [Accessed 2015].

[64]   T. Roberts, "Raw Vegetables not Always Healthier than Cooked Veggies," 20 May 2011. [Online]. Available: http://extension.missouri.edu/news/DisplayStory.aspx?N=1115.

[65]   Extension, "Cooking Methods to Preserve Nutrients in Fruits and Vegetables," 14 June 2012. [Online]. Available: http://www.extension.org/pages/24340/cooking-methods-to-preserve-nutrients-in-fruits-vegetables.

[66]   P. Van Laanen, "Safe Home Food Storage," 22 August 2002. [Online]. Available: http://travis-tx.tamu.edu/files/2010/06/Safe-Home-Food-Storage.pdf.

[67]   S. McCurdy, J. Peutz and G. Wittman, "Storing Food for Safety and Quality," University of Idaho, Washington State University, and Oregon State University, 2009.

[68]   S. Konecni and C. McClinton, SOS Gardening: Prepping Your Survival Garden for Disasters, Lafayette, Louisiana: Breakout Concepts LLC,

2013.

[69]   Clemsen Cooperative Extension, "Chemicals and Foods," February 2007. [Online]. Available: http://www.clemson.edu/extension/hgic/food/food_safety/other/hgic3860.html.

[70]   American Chemistry Council, "Plastic Packaging Resins," 2015. [Online]. Available: http://plastics.americanchemistry.com/Plastic-Resin-Codes-PDF. [Accessed 1 January 2015].

[71]   Utah State University Extension, "Ask a Specialist: Which Plastics are Safe for Food Storage," 23 July 2009. [Online]. Available: http://extension.usu.edu/htm/news-multimedia/articleID=5056.

[72]   A. Henneman and J. Jensen, "Food Reflections, Kitchen Food Safety: Bags, Bottles, and Beyond," September 2004. [Online]. Available: http://lancaster.unl.edu/food/ftsep04.htm.

[73]   J. Buffer, L. Medeiros, M. Schroeder, P. Kendall, J. LeJeune and J. Sofos, "Cleaning and Sanitizing the Kitchen Using Inexpensive Household Food-Safe Products," 2010. [Online]. Available: http://foodsafety.osu.edu/downloads/foodsafety-factsheet-sanitizing.pdf.

[74]   Partnership for Food Safety Education, 2010. [Online]. Available: http://www.fightbac.org/.

[75]   A. O'Connor, "The Claim Always Wash Your Hands With Hot Water not Cold," 12 October 2009. [Online]. Available: http://www.nytimes.com/2009/10/13/health/13real.html?_r=1&.

[76]   University of Wisconsin Cooperative Extension, "Keeping Food Safe," 2005. [Online]. Available: http://learningstore.uwex.edu/assets/pdfs/B3474.pdf.

[77] U.S. Department of Agriculture, Food Safety and Inspection Service, "The Color of Meat and Poultry," 6 August 2013. [Online]. Available: http://www.fsis.usda.gov/wps/portal/fsis/topics/food-safety-education/get-answers/food-safety-fact-sheets/meat-preparation/the-color-of-meat-and-poultry/the-color-of-meat-and-poultry/ct_index.

[78] Centers for Disease Control and Prevention, "Physical Activity and Health, The Benefits of Physical Activity," 16 February 2011. [Online]. Available: http://www.cdc.gov/physicalactivity/everyone/health/index.html.

[79] National Institutes of Health Osteoporosis and Related Bone Diseases National Resource Center, "Exercise for Your Bone Health," January 2012. [Online]. Available: http://www.niams.nih.gov/Health_Info/Bone/Bone_Health/Exercise/default.asp.

[80] B. Spencer, "Run Four Miles to Burn off just One Bottle of Coke: Scientists Call for Exercise Data to be Printed on Packaging instead of Calories," 15 October 2014. [Online]. Available: http://www.dailymail.co.uk/health/article-2796512/run-four-miles-burn-just-one-bottle-coke-scientists-call-exercise-data-printed-packaging-instead-calories.html.

[81] U.S. Department of Health and Human Services, "2008 Physical Activity Guidelines for Americans," 14 May 2015. [Online]. Available: http://www.health.gov/paguidelines/guidelines/.

[82] Harvard Medical School, "Calories Burned in 30 Minutes for People of Three Different Weights," July 2004. [Online]. Available: http://www.health.harvard.edu/newsweek/Calories-burned-in-30-minutes-of-leisure-and-routine-activities.htm.

[83] S. Knapton, "How Standing Might be the Best Anti-Aging Technique," 4 September 2014. [Online]. Available:

http://www.telegraph.co.uk/news/science/science-news/11073662/How-standing-might-be-the-best-anti-ageing-technique.html.

[84]   R. Nelson, "Just Taking Breaks from Being Sedentary May Benefit Older Adults," 6 November 2014. [Online]. Available: http://news.yahoo.com/just-taking-breaks-being-sedentary-may-benefit-older-220357995.html.

[85]   A. Sifferline, "It's Time to Pay Attention to Sleep, the New Health Frontier," 9 April 2014. [Online]. Available: http://time.com/55390/sleep-is-the-new-health-frontier/?hpt=hp_t3.

[86]   Harvard University School of Public Health, "Obesity Prevention Source, Sleep," 2015. [Online]. Available: http://www.hsph.harvard.edu/obesity-prevention-source/obesity-causes/sleep-and-obesity/. [Accessed 1 January 2015].

[87]   National Institute for Occupational Safety and Health, "Stress .....at Work," 6 June 2014. [Online]. Available: http://www.cdc.gov/niosh/docs/99-101/.

[88]   National Institutes of Health, National Institute of Mental Health, "Fact Sheet on Stress," 2015. [Online]. Available: http://www.nimh.nih.gov/health/publications/stress/index.shtml. [Accessed 1 January 2015].

[89]   R. Smith, "People Who Sleep Less than Six Hours Die Early," 5 May 2010. [Online]. Available: http://www.telegraph.co.uk/news/health/news/7677812/People-who-sleep-for-less-than-six-hours-die-early.html.

[90]   The New York Times, "Study Ties 6-7 Hours of Sleep to Longer Life," 15 February 2002. [Online]. Available: http://www.nytimes.com/2002/02/15/us/study-ties-6-7-hours-of-

sleep-to-longer-life.html.

[91]   World Health Organization, Europe, "WHO Technical Meeting on
       Sleep and Health," World Health Organization, Geneva, Switzerland,
       January 2004.

[92]   U.S. Department of Health and Human Services, National Institutes
       of Health, "Your Guide to Healthy Sleep," August 2011. [Online].
       Available:
       http://www.nhlbi.nih.gov/files/docs/public/sleep/healthy_sleep.pdf.

[93]   C. Rivette, "Research Shows Poor Sleep Impacts Weight and Health
       Risks," 26 October 2012. [Online]. Available:
       http://msue.anr.msu.edu/news/research_shows_poor_sleep_impac
       ts_weight_and_health_risks.

[94]   University of Maryland Medical Center, "Sleep Hygiene," 31 July
       2013. [Online]. Available:
       http://ummidtown.org/programs/sleep/patients/sleep-hygiene.

[95]   National Institutes of Health, National Center for Complementary
       and Integrative Health, "Sleep Disorders and Complementary Health
       Approches: What you Need to Know," April 2014. [Online]. Available:
       https://nccih.nih.gov/health/sleep/ataglance.htm.

[96]   Harvard Medical School, "Improve Sleep by Eating Right," 1
       September 2013. [Online]. Available:
       http://harvardpartnersinternational.staywellsolutionsonline.com/He
       althNewsLetters/69,L0913g.

[97]   U.S. Food and Drug Administration, "Side Effects of Sleep Drugs," 27
       February 2015. [Online]. Available:
       http://www.fda.gov/ForConsumers/ConsumerUpdates/ucm107757.
       htm.

[98]   Centers for Disease Control and Prevention, "Managing Stress," 21 May 2012. [Online]. Available: http://www.cdc.gov/features/handlingstress/.

[99]   Helpguide.org International, Harvard Medical School, "Stress Relief Guide," 2015. [Online]. Available: http://www.helpguide.org/harvard/stress-relief-guide.htm. [Accessed 1 January 2015].

[100]   American Heart Association, "Four Ways to Deal with Stress," June 2014. [Online]. Available: http://www.heart.org/HEARTORG/GettingHealthy/StressManageme nt/FourWaystoDealWithStress/Four-Ways-to-Deal-with-Stress_UCM_307996_Article.jsp.

[101]   Brandeis University, "Obesity and Stress Pack a Double Hit for Health," 22 September 2014. [Online]. Available: http://www.sciencedaily.com/releases/2014/09/140922130747.htm .

[102]   L. Schlein and M. Lipin, "Health, Environmental Hazards From Chemicals Are Rising," 5 September 2012. [Online]. Available: http://www.voanews.com/content/health_and_environmental_haz ards_from_chemicals_are_rising/1502433.html.

[103]   A. Khullar, "WHO: Air Pollution Caused One in Eight Deaths," 25 March 2014. [Online]. Available: http://www.cnn.com/2014/03/25/health/who-air-pollution-deaths/index.html?hpt=hp_t2.

[104]   Cleveland Clinic, "Household Chemicals What is in My House," 4 March 2014. [Online]. Available: http://my.clevelandclinic.org/health/healthy_living/hic_Steps_to_St aying_Well/hic_Household_Chemicals_Chart_Whats_in_my_House.

[105]   C. G. Couch and P. R. Turner, "What's in Your House," 31 October
        2013. [Online]. Available:
        http://extension.uga.edu/publications/detail.cfm?number=C1051.
        [Accessed 2015].

[106]   U.S. Environmental Protection Agency, "Pesticide Registration, Label
        Review Manual," 30 April 2015. [Online]. Available:
        http://www2.epa.gov/pesticide-registration/label-review-manual.

[107]   University of Georgia, "Green Cleaning FAQ," 2015. [Online].
        Available: http://spock.fcs.uga.edu/ext/housing/green_faq.php.
        [Accessed 1 January 2015].

[108]   Environmental Health Association of Nova Scotia, "Household
        Cleaners," 2004. [Online]. Available:
        http://www.lesstoxicguide.ca/index.asp?fetch=household. [Accessed
        2015].

[109]   M. Hefner and S. Donaldson, "What to do About Household
        Chemicals," 2015. [Online]. Available:
        http://www.unce.unr.edu/publications/files/ho/2006/fs0645.pdf.
        [Accessed 1 January 2015].

[110]   University of Missouri Extension, "Managing Household Hazardous
        Waste," 23 January 2015. [Online]. Available:
        http://extension.missouri.edu/p/WM6004.

[111]   U.S. Department of Health and Human Services, "Household
        Products Database, Health and Safety Information on Household
        Products," August 2014. [Online]. Available:
        http://householdproducts.nlm.nih.gov/.

[112]   S. Leigh and A. Mahmood, "Healthy Homes: Improving Indoor Air
        Quality," 30 June 2014. [Online]. Available:
        http://extension.missouri.edu/bsf/house/GH5001.pdf.

[113]   Montana State University Extension, "Indoor Air Quality: Home Safe Home," 2015. [Online]. Available: http://msuextensionhousing.org/resources/IndoorAirQuality.pdf. [Accessed 1 January 2015].

[114]   University of Washington, "Scented Laundry Products Emit Hazardous Chemicals through Dryer Vents," 24 August 2011. [Online]. Available: http://www.washington.edu/news/2011/08/24/scented-laundry-products-emit-hazardous-chemicals-through-dryer-vents/.

[115]   U.S. Environmental Protection Agency, "Radon, Publications and Resources," 13 May 2015. [Online]. Available: http://www.epa.gov/radon/pubs/index.html.

[116]   U.S. Environmental Protection Agency, "What Are the Six Common Air Pollutants?," 5 June 2015. [Online]. Available: http://www.epa.gov/airquality/urbanair/. [Accessed 2015].

[117]   U.S. Environmental Protection Agency, "Air Quality Index (AQI) Basics," 16 March 2015. [Online]. Available: http://airnow.gov/index.cfm?action=aqibasics.aqi. [Accessed 2015].

[118]   U.S. Environmental Protection Agency, "Water Private Wells, Frequently Asked Questions," 6 March 2012. [Online]. Available: http://water.epa.gov/drink/info/well/faq.cfm. [Accessed 2015].

[119]   B. Ross, K. Parrott and J. Woodard, "Household Water Quality, Home Water Quality Problems Causes and Treatments," 2009. [Online]. Available: http://pubs.ext.vt.edu/356/356-482/356-482_pdf.pdf. [Accessed 1 January 2015].

[120]   Centers for Disease Control and Prevention, "Common Asthma Triggers," 20 August 2012. [Online]. Available: http://www.cdc.gov/asthma/triggers.html. [Accessed 2015].

[121]   R. SoRelle, "Chronic Disease: Infectious Cause?," vol. 1998;97:2481, 1998.

[122]   L. V. Catalena and J. L. Harris, "Controlling Allergy Triggers in the Home," 2007. [Online]. Available: http://fcs.tamu.edu/housing/healthy_homes/allergy-fact-sheet.pdf.

[123]   Mayo Clinic, "Germs: Understand and Protect Against Bacteria, Viruses, and Infection," 5 May 2014. [Online]. Available: http://www.mayoclinic.org/diseases-conditions/infectious-diseases/in-depth/germs/ART-20045289.

[124]   Mayo Clinic, "Dust Mite Allergy Lifestyle and Home Remedies," 9 May 2013. [Online]. Available: http://www.mayoclinic.org/diseases-conditions/dust-mites/basics/lifestyle-home-remedies/con-20028330.

[125]   American Cleaning Institute, "Allergies and Asthma," [Online]. Available: http://www.cleaninginstitute.org/clean_living/allergies__asthma.aspx. [Accessed 1 January 2015].

[126]   Centers for Disease Control and Prevention, "Everyday Preventive Actions That Can Help to Fight Germs," 21 May 2013. [Online]. Available: http://www.cdc.gov/flu/pdf/freeresources/updated/everyday_preventive.pdf. [Accessed 2015].

[127]   Centers for Disease Control and Prevention, "Water, Sanitation, & Environmentally-related Hygiene," 30 March 2015. [Online]. Available: http://www.cdc.gov/healthywater/hygiene/.

[128]   S. Knapton, "Hand Dryers Splatter Users with Bacteria Scientists Warn," 20 November 2014. [Online]. Available: http://www.telegraph.co.uk/news/science/science-news/11243110/Hand-dryers-splatter-users-with-bacteria-scientists-

warn.html.

[129] World Health Organization, "Sexually Transmitted Infections," November 2013. [Online]. Available: http://www.who.int/mediacentre/factsheets/fs110/en/.

[130] Bioinitiative Report, 2015. [Online]. Available: http://www.bioinitiative.org/. [Accessed 1 January 2015].

[131] World Health Organization, "What are Electomagnetic Fields," 2015. [Online]. Available: http://www.who.int/peh-emf/about/WhatisEMF/en/.

[132] Federal Communications Commission, "Radio Frequency Safety FAQ," 25 June 2012. [Online]. Available: http://transition.fcc.gov/oet/rfsafety/rf-faqs.html.

[133] National Aeronautics and Space Administration, "The Electromagnetic Spectrum," March 2013. [Online]. Available: http://imagine.gsfc.nasa.gov/science/toolbox/emspectrum1.html.

[134] U.S. Food and Drug Administration, "Radiation-Emitting Products, Current Research Results," 14 October 2014. [Online]. Available: http://www.fda.gov/Radiation-EmittingProducts/RadiationEmittingProductsandProcedures/HomeBusinessandEntertainment/CellPhones/ucm116335.htm.

[135] U.S. Food and Drug Administration, "Radiation-Emitting Products, Reducing Exposure: Hands-free Kits and Other Accessories," 1 October 2014. [Online]. Available: http://www.fda.gov/radiation-emittingproducts/radiationemittingproductsandprocedures/homebusinessandentertainment/cellphones/ucm116293.htm.

[136] J. Firger, "OMG, You're Texting your Way to Back Pain," 14 November 2014. [Online]. Available: http://www.cbsnews.com/news/omg-youre-texting-your-way-to-

back-pain/.

[137]   J. Wilson, "Your Smartphone is a Pain in the Neck," 20 September
        2012. [Online]. Available:
        http://www.cnn.com/2012/09/20/health/mobile-society-neck-
        pain/index.html.

[138]   U.S. Department of Labor, "Good Working Positions," 2015. [Online].
        Available:
        https://www.osha.gov/SLTC/etools/computerworkstations/positions
        .html. [Accessed 1 January 2015].

[139]   National Institutes of Health, "Skin Health and Skin Diseases," 2008.
        [Online]. Available:
        http://www.nlm.nih.gov/medlineplus/magazine/issues/fall08/article
        s/fall08pg22-25.html.

[140]   Oregon State University, "Cutaneous Toxicity: Toxic Effects on the
        Skin," September 1993. [Online]. Available:
        http://extoxnet.orst.edu/tibs/cutaneou.htm.

[141]   R. Cornelius, "How to Use and When to Toss Makeup," 2002.
        [Online]. Available: http://www.elon.edu/e-
        web/pendulum/Issues/2004/5_6/onlinefeatures/makeup.xhtml.

[142]   U.S. Food and Drug Administration, "Use Eye Cosmetics Safely," 14
        October 2014. [Online]. Available:
        http://www.fda.gov/ForConsumers/ConsumerUpdates/ucm048943.
        htm.

[143]   National Cancer Institute, "Beauty Products and Cancer: Know the
        Facts," February 2012. [Online]. Available:
        http://www.cancer.gov/newscenter/media-
        resources/multicultural/lifelines/2012/2012-beauty-products-hl.pdf.

[144] U.S. Food and Drug Administration, "Color Additives Permitted for Use in Cosmetics," 19 September 2014. [Online]. Available: http://www.fda.gov/Cosmetics/Labeling/IngredientNames/ucm1090 84.htm. [Accessed 1 June 2015].

[145] Environmental Health Association of Nova Scotia, "Cosmetics and Personal Care," 2004. [Online]. Available: http://www.lesstoxicguide.ca/index.asp?fetch=personal.

[146] T. S. Bernard, "When Wrinkle-Free Clothing Also Means Formaldehyde Fumes," 10 December 2010. [Online]. Available: http://www.nytimes.com/2010/12/11/your-money/11wrinkle.html.

[147] American Academy of Dermatology, "Skin Cancer," 2015. [Online]. Available: https://www.aad.org/media-resources/stats-and-facts/conditions/skin-cancer.

[148] U.S. Environmental Protection Agency, "Action Steps for Sun Safety," 15 February 2015. [Online]. Available: http://www2.epa.gov/sunwise/action-steps-sun-safety.

[149] U.S. Food and Drug Administration, "Sun Safety: Save Your Skin!," 27 February 2015. [Online]. Available: http://www.fda.gov/forconsumers/consumerupdates/ucm049090.htm.

[150] U.S. Food and Drug Administration, "Think Before You Ink: Are Tattoos Safe?," 27 February 2015. [Online]. Available: http://www.fda.gov/ForConsumers/ConsumerUpdates/ucm048919.htm.

[151] J. Metcalfe, "Tattooed New Yorkers Report All Kinds of Nasty Skin Conditions," 28 May 2015. [Online]. Available: http://www.citylab.com/work/2015/05/tattooed-new-yorkers-report-all-kinds-of-nasty-skin-conditions/394304/. [Accessed 2015].

[152]   U.S. Food and Drug Administration, "FDA Taking Closer Look at Antibacterial Soap," 21 January 2015. [Online]. Available: http://www.fda.gov/forconsumers/consumerupdates/ucm378393.htm.

[153]   U.S. Food and Drug Administration, "Hand Sanitizers Carry Unproven Claims to Prevent MRSA Infections," 10 February 2015. [Online]. Available: http://www.fda.gov/forconsumers/consumerupdates/ucm251816.htm.

[154]   J. Christensen, "People Who Feel Younger at Heart Live Longer," 17 December 2014. [Online]. Available: http://www.cnn.com/2014/12/17/health/healthy-aging/index.html?hpt=hp_t4.

[155]   U.S. Department of Health and Human Services, "Thinking About Complementary and Alternative Medicine, A guide for People with Cancer," April 2005. [Online]. Available: http://www.cancer.gov/publications/patient-education/367NCINewV2.pdf. [Accessed 2015].

www.ingramcontent.com/pod-product-compliance
Lightning Source LLC
Chambersburg PA
CBHW060845280326
41934CB00007B/921